Transforming Lives with Hypnosystemic Therapy

This book provides a practise-based introductory guide for practitioners wishing to integrate hypnosystemic therapy into their services, examining its roots, principles, and methods.

Hypnosystemic therapy combines aspects of Ericksonian hypnosis, Systemic Therapy, and parts/constellation therapy into a creative awake hypnotherapy approach. This is then further consolidated in therapy or counselling. It is applied for overcoming psychological, medical, and social problems by use of conversational hypnosis mostly without trance induction. This text discusses how the intervention can be used in a variety of group and individual settings, in the treatment of diagnoses such as ADD/ADHD, allergies, hypertension, anxiety, phobias, sleeping disorders, addiction and eating disorders, and autism spectrum disorders. Chapters provide therapeutic tools in a straightforward, practical manner with examples.

Presenting therapeutic interventions in such a clear way that they can be integrated instantly into the therapeutic work of any school, this book is of particular interest to systemic therapists, behavioural therapists, and others who wish to integrate hypnotherapy knowledge into their work, but remains relevant to any mental health or allied professional.

Stefan Hammel is a German hypnotherapist and systemic therapist for children, adults, couples, and families giving live and online trainings. He is known for his storytelling, parts work, "greetings to the mind," for Ericksonian utilisation, and multilevel communication approaches.

Transforming Lives with Hypnosystemic Therapy

A Practical Guide

Stefan Hammel

Translated from German by Joanne Reynolds

Routledge
Taylor & Francis Group

LONDON AND NEW YORK

Designed cover image: © Getty Images

First published in English 2025
by Routledge
4 Park Square, Milton Park, Abingdon, Oxon, OX14 4RN

and by Routledge
605 Third Avenue, New York, NY 10158

Routledge is an imprint of the Taylor & Francis Group, an informa business

First Published in German Hypnosystemische Therapie. Das
Handbuch für die Praxis

© 2022 by Klett-Cotta, Stuttgart, www.klett-cotta.de

ISBN 978-3-608-89198-0
E-book ISBN 978-3-608-11870-4
PDF e-book ISBN 978-3-608-20554-1

The German National Library has recorded this publication in the
German National Bibliography; detailed bibliographical data are
available on the Internet at http://dnb.d-nb.de.

Library of Congress Cataloging-in-Publication Data
Names: Hammel, Stefan, author.
Title: Transforming lives with hypnosystemic therapy : a practical
guide / Stefan Hammel.
Other titles: Hypnosystemische Therapie. English
Description: Abingdon, Oxon; New York, NY: Routledge, 2024. |
Includes bibliographical references and index. | Identifiers: LCCN
2024004394 (print) | LCCN 2024004395 (ebook) | ISBN
9781032544625 (hardback) | ISBN 9781032544632 (paperback) |
ISBN 9781003425014 (ebook)
Subjects: LCSH: Hypnotism—Therapeutic use. | Systemic therapy
(Family therapy)
Classification: LCC RC497 .H363813 2024 (print) | LCC RC497
(ebook) | DDC 615.8/512—dc23/eng/20240405
LC record available at https://lccn.loc.gov/2024004394
LC ebook record available at https://lccn.loc.gov/2024004395

ISBN: 9781032544625 (hbk)
ISBN: 9781032544632 (pbk)
ISBN: 9781003425014 (ebk)

DOI: 10.4324/9781003425014

Typeset in Times New Roman
by codeMantra

Contents

PART 2
What hurts us and what heals us

PART 3
Course of therapy

Foreword

"The limits of my language mean the limits of my world", said the philosopher Ludwig Wittgenstein.[1] Language creates reality. A limiting language imposes limits on reality. The limits of imagination are the limits of possibility.

The limits of my world do not mean the limits of what is possible in the world, and they also do not mean the limits of my client's possibilities. And the limits of her language, her imagination, and her hope also do not mean the limits of her possibilities if I can succeed in expanding the limits of her world using my language and my imagination.[2]

Can it be that possibilities leading to solutions, healing, and development are lying dormant in the client, and that the only reason why she has not realised these possibilities to date is because she has not yet discovered certain physiological experiences or certain words and images? And if this is the case, how can I help her to discover this potential? Is it possible to stimulate her inner self in such a way that it makes available possibilities leading to solutions, healing, and development that had not yet been identified by her or my conscious self?

How can we expand the limits of language, the limits of imagination, and the limits of possibility in order to deliver therapeutic outcomes that are even safer, gentler, and longer-lasting, or that are achieved even faster, in order to help more people and in order to reduce the length of their suffering?

On the occasions over my years of work as a therapist when a voice inside my head has whispered to me, "That won't work", I've made it a habit to ask myself, "Are you sure? How might it work if it were to work? How does it work when it works?" I opt for the following as an experimental hypothesis: "It does work, it's just that I don't yet know how." I picture the solution that is not yet known to me like a treasure which is buried in the earth, and which I can find if I insist on the fact that the search for it is worthwhile.

Maybe our reality is what we remember and expect.

Perhaps this means that everything is in flux.

If I may, I'd like to tell you a story before we get properly started ...

Once there was a gold panner who lived in a hut by a river amidst craggy mountains. Every morning he got up, washed himself, ate a hunk of bread, got dressed in his work clothes and went to the river with his large sieve. He had already lived here for many years, and had sieved many a tonne of sand. There were days when he found a little gold, but it was seldom more than he needed to buy the absolute essentials for his day-to-day life – food, clothes, and tools. He had long dreamed of finding a large amount of gold. Yet now he guessed that this dream would probably never come true. Whenever he looked into his sieve, he mostly found nothing in it except for small pebbles that sparkled in the sun. One day an old school friend came to visit. He was a jeweller in a large city, and had made a significant fortune. He was interested in finding out for once how the gold panner lived. "Do you think you could show me how you pan for gold?" he asked his old friend. His friend hesitated and then stood up, took his sieve from the wall and went with his guest to the river. He dipped the sieve into the river, shook it from side to side and let the water run out of it. "The same as always – no gold", he sighed and looked over to his friend. "That's incredible", said his friend, who had turned pale. "Diamonds, diamonds and more diamonds!"[3]

Kaiserslautern, November 2021

Practical tips

To the best of my knowledge, I have provided sources for the interventions I have learned from colleagues. If no source is stated, I have either developed the relevant approach myself, or developed it further in such a way that it differs significantly from previously known methods. I have not generally provided sources for interventions that are assumed to be well known in expert circles. Given the large number of methods presented, omissions or errors in citing sources are possible. If any citations are missing or incorrect, I would welcome feedback so that I can cite them correctly in future editions.

All of the methods have also been trialled in a remote therapy setting using video conferencing. Any adjustments that need to be made to the procedure before its use in such a setting are explained at the relevant points in the text.

Dates and terms for training courses in hypnosystemic therapy are published on www.stefanhammel.com or can be requested under the email address: stefan.hammel@hsb-westpfalz.de. Contact data of therapists and coaches working with the methods of hypnosystemic therapy can be requested under the same address.

Notes

1 Wittgenstein 2001.
2 In the interests of readability, it is assumed throughout this book that the therapist is male, and the client is female. The principles will naturally apply regardless of their actual genders.
3 See Hammel 2012c, 88.

Part 1

Foundations

All therapy is based on the following two assumptions:

1. Everyone is equal.
2. Everyone is different.

Because everyone is equal, we can communicate.

Because everyone is different, we must communicate.

In order to understand each other, we must assume that the other person's words and body language mean the same thing that would be meant by others and by ourselves as well if we were to express ourselves in that way.

And in order to understand each other, we must on no account assume that the other person's words and body language mean the same thing that would be meant by others and by ourselves. Because if there's one thing you can rely on, it's that he means something different.[1]

Many years ago, a nurse and former pupil of Milton Erickson told me what the great man had said to her upon their parting: "If I had to choose one thing to say to you that might save you a great many detours in life, it would be this: every person on this planet of ours means something different with every word that he says."

"Words are the source of misunderstandings," said the Little Prince.[2] If we are seeking a shared basis for our communication, paying attention to someone's physiology provides a surer footing than listening to their words. Visible and audible body language is much more primeval. Some of it applies universally to communication between people (and sometimes with animals). Yet there is also room for misunderstandings, since different cultural paradigms also play a role in this connection.

If we base our actions on Assumption 1 when Assumption 2 would have proved a better fit, we can end up in a cycle of misunderstandings. It is often better to talk about "you" and "me" instead of "us". If we apply Principle 2 when Principle 1 would have proved a better fit, we can end up in a cycle of alienation and humiliation.

Othering separates men from women, indigenous peoples from colonisers, the redeemed from the unbelievers, adults from children, prison guards from prisoners, and clinicians from patients, and is accompanied by constant abasement and

DOI: 10.4324/9781003425014-1

self-abasement. A similar type of othering separates human and animal, and culture and nature. The lines along which we draw the distinction between "us" and "the others" are predominantly those that we use to separate between "good" and "evil", "right" and "wrong", "clever" and "stupid", and "healthy" and "ill".

If we think in terms of resources, opportunities, and values (the opposite of which are not negative values, but different values), then it is beneficial to construct reality together and to agree on the following: "Who am I? Who are you? Who are we? What kind of a world are we living in?" Life can then be lived as a non-zero-sum game,[3] or in other words on the basis of a "friendship" or "cooperation" model, like it says in the song: "If it's good enough for you, it's good enough for me." In contexts of this kind, the word "we" has a healing effect. Where covert or overt zero-sum games prevail, or in other words "competition" or "war" models, the word "we" has toxic qualities, and it is better to talk about "you" and "me".

In the former case it is a good idea to construct reality jointly, even if the reality that is constructed becomes neither universally true nor real as a result. In the latter case it is a good idea to distinguish between different realities, and not to insist on the construction of a shared image of reality.

From a systemic and hypnosystemic perspective, reality is in any case constructed rather than analysed. For example, Paul Watzlawick says that, "reality is what we have come to call 'reality'."[4] He provides the following explanation of what this means for therapy:

> If it is really true that our reality is always a constructed reality … what matters is replacing one construction of reality, which creates suffering and has proven to be no longer sustainable, with another which is more sustainable; nowadays that's my idea of psychotherapy.[5]

Jochen Schweitzer and Arist von Schlippe say something similar: "Reality consists of nothing more than stories,"[6] or, elsewhere:

> What we refer to as "reality" is created through dialogue, through conversation. What we see as real is what we have learned to see as real over a long process of socialisation and verbalisation. Systems construct shared realities (rather than a single reality) by way of a consensus as to how things should be seen. The shared vision of what is experienced within a system as "realities" (not a single reality) largely determines happiness or unhappiness, satisfaction or dissatisfaction.[7]

Following the same tradition, Gunther Schmidt regards the purpose of therapy as,

> offering focussing aids in the most intense and systematic way possible with a view to … searching again for potentials [that have already been stored and are available] …, finding them and activating them and then associating them into the desired life contexts in as durable a manner as possible.[8]

Allowing the client to access potentials again that existed previously but were not initially accessible to her means facilitating freedom of choice. "The central goal of all hypno-systemic interventions is to increase freedom of choice once more."[9]

It is likely that even Watzlawick no longer distinguishes strictly between therapy for the body and therapy for the mind, and this is certainly true of Schmidt. From a hypnotherapeutic and systemic point of view, the distinction between non-physical mental and non-mental physical symptoms is also largely meaningless. Hypnosystemically speaking, what is interpreted as mental, physical, social, endogenous, or exogenous is a question of the lens through which the observer is looking. The distinctions tend to be clues as to the models in the clinician's manual rather than adequate descriptions of the client's real life and suffering.

Diagnostic terms and descriptions of "pathologies" are thus also to be regarded more as clues as to clinicians' models than as descriptions of what the client is experiencing. The point is not that there is no link between the two. The point is merely that a map is not the territory it represents,[10] a passport photograph is not the individual shown, and the picture of a thing is not the thing depicted.[11] A "clinical picture" is thus also not what is going on inside a client, but merely a convention indicating what might be going on in the therapist's head when he sees the client. Similarly, a statement about whether a condition can be healed does not say anything about the client's possibilities, but merely about the clinician's possibilities, or, more accurately, the possibilities that are *known* to the clinician. It follows that prognoses do not say anything about the client's future, but merely about how things have developed on average for a number of other people who are regarded as similar in certain respects.

Diagnoses and prognoses can serve as guidance, but involve a risk. The brain always operates in the present tense. A patient's expectations about the future outlined for him in a prognosis are therefore treated by his brain in essentially the same way as memories, current perceptions, and interpretations. What was expected is what turns out to be the case. What is more, the body makes no distinction between "physical" and "mental".[12] The regulation of involuntary bodily actions and bodily reactions therefore also depends on how the patient hears, understands, and processes his prognosis. Many systemic and hypnosystemic therapists therefore avoid diagnostic terms. Concepts of illness can, however, also be acknowledged, for example with regard to the functions that they perform within the system:

> "Illness" is … not regarded as a phenomenon that is "really true", but likewise as a construct, albeit one that is often highly significant. In this connection, the construct of "illness" can in particular become a supremely important organisational element of a system, and thus from this constructivist perspective it should under no circumstances necessarily be concluded that the construct of "illness" should be unravelled in therapy in a targeted manner in order to help people in this way to free themselves from the experience of being helpless victims (something that is still a frequent practice in systemic therapy today). This seems like an eminently good idea in principle. Yet at the same time, attention

should be paid to how a different method could be used to achieve whatever "illness" might have been working towards in an (unconsciously) desired manner within a system, e.g. greater cohesion within the system. Otherwise the attempt to unravel concepts of illness might be experienced as a threat and meet resistance in response.[13]

Concepts of illness can also be used (or utilised) for the client's health and well-being. Taking diagnostic terms as a starting point, the model of disease is visualised in such a way that the solutions implied by this model (e.g. the body's good intentions) generate ideas of how therapy or a certain behaviour by the client might reduce suffering (limitations) and promote well-being (expanded opportunities).[14]

Notes

1 "All is one, all is different." Pascal 1961, 67 (*Pensées* 125). The philosophical and theological concept of the indivisible one and all (*hen kai pan*) requires the paradoxical juxtaposition of different elements. The axiom of simultaneous unity and variety also applies to the hypnosystemic understanding of identity. Every actualised "I" conceals many possible ones.

2 The original quote is: "Le langage est source de malentendus." Saint-Exupéry 2017, 70.

3 For further details of (non-)zero-sum games, see Watzlawick et al. 1967, 130, 227, 285.

4 Watzlawick et al. 2011, 130 *passim*.

5 Paul Watzlawick, in: Maurer 2021. See Muffler 2015, 21: "Hypno-systemic … therapy [provides] … support in terms of altering the construction of reality..."

6 Schlippe & Schweitzer 1996, 40. See Groß & Popper 2020, 76: "Our internal images create our realities."

7 Schlippe & Schweitzer 1996, 89.

8 Schmidt 2005, 67 *et seqq.*

9 Ibid., 67.

10 "A map is not the territory it represents, but, if correct, it has a similar structure to the territory, which accounts for its usefulness." Korzybski 1994, 58.

11 The problem of confusing the image of the thing with the thing itself is illustrated by René Magritte's painting "Ceci n'est pas une pipe" (This Is Not A Pipe), see www.publicdelivery.org/magritte-not-a-pipe. Cf. Pascal: "What an empty thing is painting, which makes us admire the copies of things which we do not admire at all in the original!" (Pascal 1961, 65, *Pensées* 116). If a thing must be depicted within us in order to be perceived, when do we see the thing or the person itself? What (or whom) are we reacting to?

12 The construct of mind/body separation takes place in the observer's thoughts, and has no scientific basis, but instead results from the Platonic worldview.

13 Schmidt 2005, 54.

14 Narrative reframings for most psychiatric diagnoses can be found in Hammel 2016a.

Chapter 1

What is hypnosystemic therapy?

Hypnosystemic therapy is a term used to refer to types of talking therapy that combine elements of systemic therapy, Ericksonian hypnotherapy and also often parts work and structural constellations[1] in an active–alert dialogue. The term "hypnosystemic" was introduced by Gunther Schmidt in 1980 or thereabouts. Schmidt lists the following reasons for the integration of the Ericksonian and systemic approaches in a *single* concept:

> The starting point for both is the idea that all life processes should be examined with a view to potentially describing patterns. Both understand living systems as self-organising, autopoietic systems …
>
> Both … start from an almost identical understanding of how change can happen (through the emergence of differences in previously prevalent patterns).[2]

The amalgamation of approaches also makes sense because their development was closely intertwined from the outset. Schmidt refers in this connection to the fact that, "for many years, almost all of the key interventions within the systemic approach have been borrowed from Ericksonian hypnotherapy."[3]

The systemic approach was popularised in Germany from 1974 onwards by the Munich Family College (Gaby Moskau, Gerd Müller), the Munich Institute for Integrative Family Therapy (Carole Gammer, Martin Kirschenbaum), the Weinheim Institute run by Maria Bosch,[4] the Mannheim College of Social Affairs (Elisabeth Nader), and, most famously, the Heidelberg Group around Helm Stierlin.

These individuals were in close communication with Salvador Minuchin and the Milan Group around Mara Selvini Palazzoli. Both groups were in contact with the Californian Palo Alto Group including Paul Watzlawick, Jay Haley, Virginia Satir, and others, who in turn were in close communication with Milton Erickson and Gregory Bateson.

Paul Watzlawick, John Weakland, and Richard Fisch provided a theoretical foundation for systemic therapy by linking its practice to the axioms of group theory (Evariste Galois), logical type theory (Alfred Whitehead and Bertrand Russell)[5] and systems theory (Niklas Luhmann and others).

DOI: 10.4324/9781003425014-2

Gunther Schmidt, who belonged to the Heidelberg Group, became acquainted with Milton Erickson in Arizona and, like a number of other colleagues,[6] brought the inspiration he had gained from Erickson's work back with him to Germany.

In the USA, Virginia Satir developed family therapy concepts and the family sculpture method, which she also taught to German colleagues.

Her method – which she popularised in a modified form as "family roles" – became known to Bert Hellinger in Munich. There was later a break between Hellinger and the majority of his colleagues working in the systemic tradition. After some years had passed, the relationship between those working in the constellation tradition and system therapists eased, with the exception of Hellinger, who was considered apart, as attested to by the book title "Constellation work revisited ... in a post-Hellinger era?"[7] In the systemic and hypnosystemic context, Gunthard Weber in Wiesloch as well as Insa Sparrer and Matthias Varga von Kibéd in Munich (among others) teach constellation work techniques. At the same time, they are in regular contact with Schmidt and other colleagues working in the hypnosystemic tradition. In the field of parts work, colleagues from the hypnosystemic school maintain close links with representatives of ego state therapy such as Kai Fritzsche and Woltemade Hartman, among others.

What role does the Hammelian form of therapy play in this story?

A colleague who had read the manuscript wrote the following:

In my view, what is new is ... the further development of spatialisation techniques. The spatialisation of life's possibilities and options for history taking and therapy. The bidding of farewell to parts. The greetings ... Working in a hypnotherapeutic style, you take a respectful and appreciative approach by transforming what is already available in a wholly exceptional and remarkable manner and adding something new to it.

He wanted to know what I thought: "What is the essence of Stefan Hammel, what are the concepts that are original and unique to Stefan Hammel?"[8]

• One of my contributions has been to lend a narrative and dialogic form to hypnosis-based work. This includes outlining the adjustments that are needed to use hypnosis in conditions experienced as active–alert at least as effectively as in a deep trance.[9] This involves the development of narrative hypnosystemic work as a form of therapy, or in other words the skilful use of metaphors and paradigmatic stories as well as the transformation of the client's burdensome life stories into restorative self-narratives. This includes the first ever description of an overall concept integrating the mechanisms of action and creative possibilities of therapeutic stories.[10]

• A further achievement that is worth mentioning is the development of therapeutic modelling as a new form of therapy. This is a radically flexibilised yet simultaneously rules-based form of interaction with personified life possibilities, which – in keeping with the precepts of Ericksonian therapy – are dissociated, associated, and narratively transformed until as far as possible a symptom-free state is achieved.[11]

- Working with therapeutic greetings is an entirely new method.[12] It is a particularly effective, rapid, and versatile procedure aimed at stimulating changes in the client's involuntary reactions, and a form of ultra-short hypnosis based on Ericksonian forms of communication.
- Another contribution to the field is raising greater awareness among therapists of certain elements of Ericksonian hypnotherapy that had receded into the background, such as the use of anecdotes and other narrative elements, therapeutic double binds, multilevel communication and various different forms of utilisation.
- To this can be added the integration of spiritual concepts into therapeutic work in such a form that the content can also be accepted by therapists and clients with differing or uncertain religious convictions.
- A final contribution is the development and description of hundreds of effective individual interventions, both for specific therapeutic situations and also, in a generalisable form, for an arbitrary number of different applications.

Mention should also be made of the following contributions to the expert discussion:

- the first and currently the only book on utilisation as the central approach of Ericksonian therapy,[13]
- the first comprehensive presentation of therapeutic multilevel communication as the second central element of Milton Erickson's work,[14]
- the book you have in your hands, as the first major coherent outline of hypnosystemic therapy.

There's a further point I'd like to make at this stage, if I may; hypnosystemic therapy is in effect not a "specific method", but can instead be described as a therapeutic attitude that gives rise to a broad spectrum of methods. The following consensus is presupposed by Schmidt:

> that "the" systemic therapy or counselling does not exist, but that its story is characterised by the manifold and simultaneous blossoming of many differentiations of the principles.[15]

The same applies to hypnosystemic therapy: the approaches used by therapists working within this tradition cannot be described as a uniform construct, and still less as a "school". Instead, it is a range of approaches that are related and in dialogue with each other.[16]

This book too does not describe *the only* hypnosystemic approach. Instead, it outlines a spectrum of possibilities for hypnosystemic therapy and presents an interpretation of what defines hypnosystemic work.

Notes

1 Schmidt refers to the following as influences: "body therapy methods such as psychodrama, transactional analysis and Gestalt therapy, but also behavioural therapy." Schmidt 2005, 9. Jochen Peichl makes the following thought-provoking point: "We must somehow assemble Milton Erickson's hypnotherapy, systemic thinking and therapeutic work with parts into a single structure that does not creak too much at the seams." Peichl 2019, 9 *et seq.*

2 Schmidt 2004, 38 et seq., Schmidt 2005, 7 *et seq.*

3 Schmidt 2004, 39, see Schmidt 2005, 10.

4 Satir 2018, 11 *et seq.*, 48.

5 Watzlawick et al. 2011. Foundational approaches for psychotherapy that were drawn from the field of communication sciences can be found in such early works as Watzlawick et al. 1967.

6 Wilhelm Gerl, Alida Jost-Peter, Hans-Ulrich Schachtner, Bernd Schmid, Peter Nemetschek, and Burkhard Peter also became familiar with Erickson's work by observing it themselves.

7 Weber et al. 2005.

8 Klaus Haasis, email dated 23 July 2021.

9 See Chapter 2, Section "Factors affecting therapy", Hammel 2019a, 8 *et seqq.*

10 Hammel 2019a.

11 See Chapter 2, Section on the role of psychodrama, constellation work and parts' work, Chapter 7, Section on history taking using life opportunities and Chapter 8, Section "Therapeutic modelling", Hammel 2019b, Hammel et al. 2020, 74 *et seqq.*

12 See Chapter 8, Section "Therapeutic greetings", Hammel 2020.

13 Hammel 2011, see Hammel 2012b.

14 Hammel 2014a.

15 Schmidt 2004, 16.

16 The boundaries between those who are working "hypnosystemically" and those who are not are blurred. In addition to Gunther Schmidt's approach and my concepts, models and procedures developed by the following are also associated with the term: Peter Allemann, Reinhold Bartl, Hiltrud Bierbaum-Luttermann, Wiltrud Brächter, Daniel Dietrich, Jean-Otto Domanski, Martina Gross, Philip Häublein, Peter Hain, Ina Hullmann, Roland Kachler, Andreas Kollar, Anne Lang, Werner Leeb, Dorothea Leichsenring, Ortwin Meiss, Manuela Mey, Cordula Meyer-Erben, Anne Müller, Elvira Muffler, Siegfried Mrochen, Andrea Niedrist, Michael and Barbara Nigitz-Arch, Jochen Peichl, Tilman Peschke, Peter Pfeifer, Vera Popper, Mechthild Reinhard, Claudia Reinicke, Sabine Rösler, Hanne Seemann, Karin Sautter-Ott, Susy Signer-Fischer, Vera Starker, Antonio de Stefano, Peter Stimpfle, Bernhard Trenkle, Martin Weckenmann, Ute Zander-Schreindorfer, Silvia Zanotta and Reinhold Zeyer (non-exhaustive list). A synopsis of different models can be found at www.hager-katharina.at/grundlagen.

Chapter 2

Basic assumptions

I intend to expand below on a number of ideas that will serve as a basis for the more detailed explorations that follow.

The body and the mind are a *single* system. All bodily experiences are permeated by intellectual and psychological influences and impacts, including social, biographical, and family biographical influences and impacts. The question of whether an ailment has a physical or a psychological cause makes little or no sense when viewed from this perspective. More precisely, the answer to this question does not describe a reality within the system, but instead provides a clue as to the lens (mental or physical) through which the audience is viewing this individual's ailment.

Everything that is somatic is also psychological, and everything that is psychological is also somatic.[1] Schmidt uses the term "somatopsychological" in this connection.[2]

If the term "psychological" primarily refers to the sphere of thoughts and emotions, what then are thoughts? And what are emotions?

Thinking is simulated perception in sequences, and takes place in stories. The underlying sensory perceptions are interlinked in different ways and to different degrees. Some people "see" sounds and tastes, for example (synaesthesia). When we talk about thinking, we are typically referring to one of the following three or four procedures – or to a combination of them, because it is likely that all of the different variants come into play in all individuals, with differing priorities.

The first case relates to simulated *visual* experience, or in other words internal video or image sequences. Reference can alternatively be made to daydreams, with a distinction between those that relate to the past (memory), the present (interpretation of current perception), the future (expectation, often as hope or fear), or completely fictional matters.

The second case relates to simulated *auditory* perception in the form of internal monologues. Sometimes we experience ourselves predominantly as the listener of spoken content (and experience a second inner self or another person as the speaker in this connection), sometimes we experience ourselves predominantly as the speaker (addressing ourselves or an imagined other), and sometimes we

DOI: 10.4324/9781003425014-3

experience ourselves as engaging in a dialogue, by alternating between the roles of listener and speaker.

Some people with mainly *kinaesthetic* access to themselves and to the world experience their thoughts as being formed out of bodily feelings and bodily reactions, or in other words penetrating into their consciousness out of their physiological experience.

Certain individuals have "ticker tape synaesthesia", where they visualise the words spoken by inner voices passing by in front of their inner eye; this means that they "read thoughts" to some extent, which is a *verbal and visual* variant of thinking.

Others have purely verbal associations with the term "thinking", which means that they concentrate on the second variant and distinguish thinking from dreaming. As I see it, thinking is the form of dreaming that incorporates verbal language.

And **emotions**? If we observe what happens while we are experiencing and expressing an emotion, the main thing we notice will be bodily reactions. This includes involuntary muscular movements, tensing and relaxing of the muscles, changes in breathing, cardiac activity and therefore also blood flow, trembling, vibrating or pulsing movements, different bodily sensations, changes in mucous membranes, activation of the lacrimal glands, and many more. Emotions are interlinked bodily reactions whose interaction is not assigned to the respective bodily parts, but experienced as a reaction to external, mostly socially constructed events.

We react by means of emotions to changes in our sense of safety, belonging, and importance within our social system ("herd"), and to expected or actual losses and damage to our safe place ("territory", "home", "private life").

As I see it, the list of emotions includes loneliness, anger and annoyance, fear and timidity, sadness, disgust, reluctance and horror or dread, sentiment and feeling, shame and guilt, as well as joy, in each case with their various facets. Goodwill and aversion or envy can also be listed as combinations of emotions and desires (granting someone something good or bad or begrudging them something good). Mention can also be made of gratitude and resentment as combinations of emotions and memory, and optimism and despondency as combinations of emotions and expectation.

Emotions such as fear or sadness also occur if the survival or integrity of our innermost territory – the body – is at risk. Disgust on the other hand is the fear of bodily orifices. People are disgusted if they experience or are afraid that something might penetrate (via wounds or natural bodily orifices) into their body against their will, or if they identify with another person who is in a similar situation.

Thoughts and emotions are experienced – or in other words perceived – bodily. In the case of thoughts, visual and auditory *perception* is in the foreground for most people, at least in a state of (or close to) waking consciousness; in the case of emotions, it is bodily feelings and bodily reactions. In the world of our dreams (including the current construed perception), sight, hearing, touch, and the other senses are a *single* network. Thoughts and emotions are therefore two parts of a whole, with an emphasis on different sensory channels: if we think, we also feel, and if we feel, we also think.

Sensory perception therefore serves as the interface – for the most part via the imagination as a network of simulated sensory impressions – between what we regard as physical and what we experience mentally.

Our immune system also has sensory channels which, just like our sight, hearing, and smell, sound out the potential of opportunities and dangers relating to incoming stimuli. Like the other senses, it learns, expects, and remembers and creates helpful or erroneous links between stimulus and reaction. Social or territorial experiences that are associated with excessive stress sometimes cause trigger reactions that are identical to traumatic stimulus-reaction patterns. Medically speaking, many of the trigger patterns controlled by the immune system can be describe as autoimmune diseases. It is telling that reference is made to "systematic desensitisation" when treating both phobias and allergies. It would appear that not only the therapy, but also the disorder treated is essentially the same, and it is simply the case that sometimes (in the case of most diagnosed phobias) the visual perception system sends out a false alarm, and other times a corresponding error is made from an immunological perspective.[3] Alongside the conscious channels of perception, there are therefore also channels that remain unconscious but behave in an analogous fashion. As I see it, all therapeutic interventions that work on phobias and traumatic triggers also work on allergies, and vice versa.[4] The connection also becomes apparent if we ask patients suffering from allergies: "How long has that been going on for you? And what else was happening at the time?"

Every perception requires interpretation, and it goes without saying that things which are perceived and interpreted are subject to error in the sense of over-interpretation, under-interpretation and misinterpretation.[5] It is becoming increasingly clear that our senses do not so much analyse reality as construct reality, which is why we might say that, "reality *is* what we have come to *call* 'reality'."[6] "Reality" is a culturally developed concept and an outcome of jointly interpreted perceptions rather than their primary source. If we think that we are analysing what we (or our ancestors and the society in which we interpret our environment) previously created, we enter into cycles of self-corroborating assumptions. A distinction can be made between the reality constructed by individuals – potentially regarded by others as paranoid – and the "consensus reality"[7] of societal majorities or conviction-based communities. The latter generate plausibility in a variety of different ways, for example standardised experimental settings, religious revelation, authority legitimated by the family or the state or trust in the information-sharing structures of media bubbles. If a group or an individual does not accept the preconditions laid down by the others with a view to creating plausibility (which is typically based on reciprocity), a shared reality cannot be established, as in the case of therapy with patients diagnosed as suffering from "mania". It is often the case that effective work can, however, be carried out if the therapist accepts the reality constructed by his client and ensures that everything he says remains within the constraints of this reality.

2.1 Assumptions and attitudes from hypnotherapy

Hypnosystemic therapy uses concepts from hypnotherapy, in particular from the tradition of Milton Erickson. By way of contrast to traditional hypnotherapy, hypnosystemic work does not typically use formal trance induction or induce deep trances. The style of therapy is largely based on dialogue, and the therapist–client encounter is based on a willingness to engage in a partnership as equals.

Milton Erickson's attitude was characterised by curiosity, love, respect, and the acceptance of everything brought to him by the client. This attitude, as well as his belief that the client already has everything she needs, led to a shift, albeit one that probably applied less to Erickson himself and more to those working in the post-Erickson era: the client is on an equal ranking with the therapist. This means that the therapist has nothing to hide from the client. There are no techniques that must remain a "black box" from the client. Moral or pathological judgements have no place in a respectful, skills-oriented approach. This also means that the client's skills and the therapist's skills combine together to create the solution experience sought by the client.

Milton Erickson was extremely keen on interventions. He regularly took the lead with his therapeutic inputs. He followed his patients in another way, however:

> Each person is a unique individual. Hence, psychotherapy should be formulated to meet the uniqueness of the individual's needs, rather than tailoring the person to fit the Procrustean bed of a hypothetical theory of human behavior.[8]

Erickson's manner of speaking during hypnosis sessions was conversational rather than imperative, and it also did not resemble the manner typically used for formal hypnosis. It was often not clear to participants when the actual "hypnosis" started, or whether what was happening at that particular moment in time was already "hypnosis" or still "hypnosis".

Hypnosystemic therapy builds on this style of conversation and develops it further by inviting clients to engage in active–alert imaginative experiments. It dispenses with trance rituals and stimulates dissociative processes through the use of voice and body language, through signal words that are casually dropped into the conversation, through the deliberate choice of appropriate grammatical constructions and through intentionally selected parables and anecdotes. It retains the key fundamental concepts from hypnosis work. I'd like to provide a brief explanation with reference to a number of basic concepts.

Hypnosis is the deliberate induction of trance phenomena using rapport and suggestion. Hypnotic processes are everyday processes. The phenomena we typically regard as hypnosis also occur when we are reading an exciting book: anaesthesia (freedom from pain), amnesia (ignoring ambient noise), negative and positive hallucinations (not seeing individual letters, perceiving things that are not there), altered perception of time, catalepsy (stiffening of the body), automatic movements (turning the pages) and much more.

Trance is not a specific state; instead, "the term 'trance' encompasses all experience-based processes in which involuntary experience is dominant."[9] This means states where what is experienced is subject to noticeable dissociation (i.e. ignoring or splitting), association (i.e. linking or identification), or transformation (i.e. gradual change, for example in internal films).

"Trance phenomena", such as the inability to move a body part (catalepsy)[10] or anaesthesia[11] can also be achieved without inducing a trance.

Not every trance is relaxing, and not every trance is desirable. States of acute trauma, panic attacks, depression, psychosis, and physical crises are also associated with trances, but this does not mean that they are beneficial or predominantly pleasant states. In a therapeutic context, Schmidt distinguishes between problem trances and wish or solution trances.[12] Problem trances result from the focusing of attention on matters that are stressful and that restrict possibilities, and solution trances result from the focusing of attention on matters that are freeing and that open up possibilities, as well as on opportunities, resources, and skills.

Suggestion is the directing of attention. To put it another way, suggestion is the stimulation of change in another person's experience, generated either consciously or unconsciously. Suggestion brings about change in terms of perceptions and interpretations, desires and aversions, beliefs, and impulses to act.

One cannot not suggest,[13] one can only be unaware of one's own suggestions. Suggestions can be both verbal and non-verbal. What we omit (in line with or contrary to expectations) also has a suggestive effect.

Any form of communication is involuntarily suggestive. This is at any rate true if we assume that, "every human experience is fundamentally [to be interpreted as] the outcome and expression of the focusing of attention,"[14] and that this focusing of attention is controlled reciprocally, as part of the interplay of communication, through the contributions made by the partners (or opponents). Gunther Schmidt uses the term "very strong invitations" in this connection. Since we need to imagine things in order to understand them, some of these invitations ("Don't think about the colour blue!") are so compelling that the concept of reciprocal control ("leading") is also plausible, however.

The effectiveness of suggestion (or hypnotherapy) does not depend specifically on the depth of the trance or a certain type of trance, but on the fact that an arrangement is established within which the client internally agrees to the suggestions that are offered. Formal trance inductions are only one of a range of different methods for promoting the client's agreement with the effectiveness of therapy.[15] Placebos often work extremely well even in the absence of a trance, for example.

When a trance is stimulated, only the sphere of experience in which objections might be raised to the outcome of therapy is decoupled from the sphere in which therapeutic learning takes place. In order to achieve the same outcome in an active–alert dialogue, relevance and plausibility are constructed for what is suggested.

The relevance and plausibility of objections that stand in the way of the success of therapy are accordingly deconstructed. No logical plausibility is required in this connection. A perceived, intuitive plausibility is sufficient.[16]

Closer examination of the **focusing of attention** makes it possible to describe the physiological processes involved in a more differentiated manner than when using the term "trance".[17] We can outline multidimensional landscapes of attention in which aspects of experience associated to differing extents with the ego experience are depicted as mountains and those dissociated from it as valleys. If we want to incorporate the transformative element (or in other words the change in attention over a certain period of time), we must effectively use a 3D animation to show how the mountains and valleys form and shift over the course of a sequence of therapy.[18]

We talk about **patterns** if the focusing of attention – by individuals or parts of a system – is characterised by repetition. Certain patterns can be described quasi-statically, as bodily snapshots (patterns of experience, e.g. trigger reactions), and others more dynamically, as a succession of different stages of a process (behavioural and interaction patterns, escalation spirals). When describing patterns, we can adopt a wide-angled focus by considering the systemic interaction of all those directly involved, society as a whole, and other environmental factors, or a narrow-angled focus by examining internal communication in daydreams, internal monologues, or bodily reactions.[19]

Rapport is the involuntary joint construction of reality. This includes congruences in terms of physical behaviour, manner of speaking and voice, verbal expression, the interpretation of current situations and content of speech (including worldview), aesthetic preferences, values, and much more. The metaphor of a "shared wavelength", the term "fusion of horizons" as coined by Gadamer or the experience of a "sense of togetherness" can be used to clarify the meaning of rapport.

The term **"yes set"** is used to refer to a series of statements to which the listener can be expected to respond in agreement. Each statement of this kind and each agreement increases the likelihood that the following statement will also be answered in the affirmative, even if it would probably not be accepted in a different context.

Pacing means taking as a basis the behaviour and experience of one's counterpart, and implies the building of and increase in rapport. We can pace our counterpart's breathing, body posture, manner of speaking, vocabulary, thinking, and every other manifestation of life by aligning ourselves with his behaviour. Pacing is crucially important with a view to meeting the client in her initial experience (her "problem trance"), promoting trust and achieving consensus. A complex, multilayered experience in the client can be countered by means of analogous communication on the part of the therapist (ambivalence pacing[20]).

Leading means the shaping or joint shaping of a common experience, and implies a suggestive behaviour. Leading is crucially important with a view to bringing the client closer to her target experience; one could also talk about promoting a solution trance. Like pacing, leading can be achieved both verbally and non-verbally.

The terms "pacing" and "leading" were introduced by the Neuro-Linguistic Programming (NLP) founders Richard Bandler and John Grinder in order to describe what Milton Erickson referred to as "establishing a yes set".

Utilisation is the use ...

- of elements of the initial situation to achieve the target situation,
- of what is already working for what is not yet working, and
- of the familiar and incontrovertible to achieve the desired results.

Utilisation is characterised by an appreciation for everything that the client and the therapeutic situation presents us with, and a willingness to use all of it.

Utilisation is therefore an attitude of valuing, thinking, and searching, and a behavioural orientation.[21] It is not restricted to a particular technique, form of intervention, or strategy for action.

In Milton Erickson's opinion, the therapist's task is accordingly, "an initial acceptance of the patient's presenting behavior by the operator, however seemingly adverse that presenting behavior may appear to be in the clinical situation." As part of this process, "the subject's own attitudes, thinking, feeling, and behavior, and aspects of the reality situation [are] variously employed."[22] In a certain sense, the campaigning slogan of utilisation is, "value everything and use everything!", whereby "value" might not always mean "like" in this connection, but does always mean "respect".

Multilevel communication is a way of taking in information and self-communication which perceives and categorises interlocutors' manifestations of life at many different sensory and linguistic levels synchronously. What is offered by the therapist (the deconstruction of problem experiences, the construction of solution experiences and the transformation of problem experiences into solution experiences) is accordingly conveyed on many channels synchronously, both verbally and non-verbally. This can be compared to the coordinatory efforts of someone driving through heavy traffic or playing the piano in a band, both of whom integrate many actions and sensory perceptions and take decisions in rapid succession – both intuitively and close to the conscious mind (accessible to reflection) – governing how they act and react.

When starting out with multilevel communication, it should be remembered that what matters is the choice of words together with their value judgements and connotative fields, the syntax, the use of tenses, the use of indicative, subjunctive, imperative, and question forms, the use of affirmations, imperatives and questions, anecdotes and parables, and the dramaturgy of spoken words in general. On a visible and non-verbal level, attention is paid to facial expressions and gestures, to the nature of movement, to changes in skin colouration, breathing and other involuntary bodily reactions; on an audible and non-verbal level, attention is paid to the voice, the manner of speaking, and flow of speech, to any clearing of the throat and to other sounds made by the body. Other important factors include observations regarding clothing, personal care, courtesies, and other customs.[23]

2.1.1 Factors affecting therapy

When are therapeutic interventions effective? When are they potentially less so?

The researcher Matthew Lieberman has discovered that the mind finds its way back to emotional equilibrium in three main ways:

1. we identify what we are feeling (*putting emotions into words*),
2. we think differently about the situation (*reinterpretation*),
3. we think about something else ... (*distraction*).

Another researcher, James Coan, has added another piece to the puzzle of the options available to a mind that wishes to find peace again:

4. the actual or imagined presence of an individual who is thought to like us (*accompaniment*).[24]

Therapeutic interventions that take these factors into consideration are likely to help reduce and (where applicable) dispel emotional stresses and the associated physical and social symptoms relatively quickly, safely, and durably.

Based on my observations, the following principles apply to the effectiveness of therapeutic interventions and are fundamentally in line with these outcomes:

1. The more perceptible an intervention, the more effective it is.

The more the therapy can be seen, heard, felt, and made tangible to the senses, the more easily available the outcome is later as a memory from which expectation and experiences can be generated.[25] The following are therapeutically effective:

- simulated perception (imagination),
- the use of visible objects and spatial arrangements,
- symbolic actions,[26]
- changes that can be experienced by the body.

The corollary of this is the following:

- The greater the extent to which the therapy is experienced spatially, the more effective it is.
- Therapy calls for experience, drama, and emotion. (Conversely, suffering is not an absolute prerequisite for the therapeutic process, and can even damage it.)
- The more concrete the terms and scenes used in the solution context, the more easily the client can process what she has heard.
- The more abstract the terms and scenes used in the problem context, the less likely it is that the problem in the client's imagination will inhibit the finding of solutions.

2. The more relevant and plausible an intervention appears, the more effective it is.

What is relevant is what fits in with the client's system of values, or in other words what she regards as good, useful and likely to strengthen her and expand her opportunities, or to protect her in an obvious manner against danger, suffering, loss, or negative impacts of any kind whatsoever.

What is plausible is what is experienced by the client as coherent, or in other words what does not provoke an objection. The following types of plausibility can be identified …

- logical plausibility: "Scientists have discovered that …"
- emotional plausibility: "It needs a good kicking!"
- experienced plausibility: "You look relieved." "You can see this door, right?"
- narrative plausibility: "Like all dung beetles, he loved dung."
- intuitive plausibility: "Watch out! I'm suffering from infectious health."

The basis for the plausibility of therapeutic interventions is irrelevant. Any kind of perceived plausibility and relevance to the client's life ensures that suggestions are implemented. The question as to whether a trance is involved is of comparatively minor importance. It is sufficient to formulate what is said in such a way that the client is not expected to respond in the negative, regardless of the reasons why.

3. The fewer the client's objections to the therapy at the end of the session, the more stable the outcome.

To put it in a formula:

The client's feeling of plausibility regarding the progress of therapy
minus
her feeling of plausibility regarding objections/the continuation of what existed before
equals
the value achieved in terms of the stability of the therapeutic outcome.

The client's conscious or unconscious objections to the efficacy of therapy are *the* factor that limits effectiveness. They function as counter-suggestions that invalidate part of the therapeutic outcome. From time to time, external sceptics are more powerful than internal ones. If a child's father or mother, a doctor, a therapist or another authority figure hints or explicitly says that the therapy might not work, this often has devastating consequences.

At the latest towards the end of the session, it is a good idea to spend a certain amount of time and care constructing a high level of perceived plausibility for the long-lasting nature of what has been achieved and deconstructing the plausibility of any objections raised by the client or her environment against the validity and longevity of the outcome.[27]

4. The more the first session is experienced as effective by the client and the more confident she therefore is when embarking upon the second session, the faster the entire course of therapy will be.

If the first therapy session has delivered a remarkably large number of outcomes from the client's perspective, she will expect the same for the second and typically then also experience that this is what happens.

This means that everything that is likely to generate less therapeutic change should be avoided, in particular at the start of therapy, and conversely everything that is likely to generate a lot of change should be implemented.

It also means that during the first session it is not a good idea to allow the client to talk for any longer than absolutely necessary about her problem, to incorporate a long history-taking phase, or to explain therapeutic concepts to her. Instead, this time can be used to allow her to try out new perspectives that make a helpful difference to her life.

It is of course crucially important for the client to feel seen, welcome, and valued, but therapy will be more effective if this can be achieved without spending any extra time on it. Major contributions to this end are made by the therapist's posture, facial expressions, and gestures, his voice and manner of speaking, his choice of words and use of courtesies, references to the good intention of his approach, and questions about how the client feels about it.

5. Healing is the result of defocusing and refocusing.

Clients' concerns are often very easy to comprehend: doing badly at school, arguments with a partner, compulsive rumination. Concrete questions can be asked about concrete concerns: "Since when has that been a problem? What else was going on at the time?", "Had you experienced something similar to the stress back then earlier in your life, perhaps as a child?", and "Did your parents and grandparents experience something similar?"

In the process of answering questions similar to the above, the client **defocuses** from her *current* reliving of older stress reactions and **refocuses** on *earlier* triggers that often provide a better explanation than current events of why she is now reacting in this way (and reacting so violently).

By gaining insight into the fact that she is able to protect herself against the old stresses but no longer needs to do so, she *defocuses* from the earlier events and *refocuses* on the initial situation with a relaxed new perspective. If the therapist is treating several clients at once (e.g. a couple), it is helpful to offer a perspective of this kind to all those involved.

6. Healing is the result of re-experiencing paralysed emotions in a regulated fashion.

If people regularly – and particularly in childhood – experience an inability to express their emotions because they are otherwise threatened with severe sanctions (such as verbal humiliation or physical violence), or because no one is interested in how they feel (e.g. caregivers' physical absence or lack of interest, dissociation through addiction, depression, or grief), they often develop problems in terms of perceiving or expressing emotions. Clients often speak about loneliness, abandonment, or an unfathomable deep anxiety in this context. Difficulties in terms of feeling and expressing certain emotions or all emotions are often associated with reduced bodily awareness, and in some cases also with problems relating to visual and acoustic perception. The phenomenon of paralysed, numbed, or blocked emotions plays a particular role in the context of traumatic stresses.[28] Psychological phenomena such as depression, mania, addiction, and psychosis can be interpreted as an attempt by the body to numb an overwhelming pain so that this pain can be dealt with.[29] Similarly, many physical symptoms can be traced back to periods of emotional overload.[30] To put it another way, strong emotions that are not expressed over an extended period of time are frequently transformed into physical symptoms as the result of an experience of existential threat.

A factor of decisive importance for the effectiveness of therapy is the extent to which the client is able, without becoming overloaded, to experience and express emotions that she has at times been unable to experience or only able to experience in an extreme form. It is sufficient to perceive the individual emotions jointly and to recognise them as appropriate in their context. A high level of emotional intensity is not required for healing.[31]

2.1.2 The cycle of memory and expectation

The terms "past", "present", and "future" refer to our location in physical time. The conundrum of time is one that has occupied philosophers from time immemorial and results from the conceptual commingling of physical time and our biological experience of time. For our purposes, we can limit our considerations to the following.

Biologically constituted beings always live in the "now". *The past is memory in the now. The present is construed perception in the now. The future is expectation in the now, typically realised as hope or fear. Everything that happens in the now can influence and be influenced, and can benefit and be of benefit.*

This "now" denotes the temporal self-positioning of our perceiving mind in the same way as the "here" denotes its spatial self-positioning, the "is" (by way of contrast to the "would be" or the "is said to be") denotes its self-positioning with a view to the realised possibilities and the "I" denotes its self-positioning with a view to other persons or possible ways of being a person.

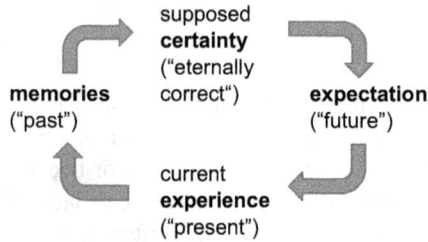

Figure 2.1 The cycle of memory and expectation

Memory, expectation, and experience are simulated perception, or in other words internal films in our head, including the associated bodily sensations and bodily reactions.

Expectations are made from memories – good expectations (hopes) from good memories, and bad expectations (fears) from bad memories. What we expect becomes what we get more often than we think, and an expectation becomes an experience.

What is the effect of an expectation,

- that we will slip over on black ice?
- that the placebo is a medication that will help?
- that our mind will go blank in the exam?
- that the boss will say no?
- that hypnosis helps?

A bad memory thus becomes a bad expectation, which becomes a bad experience, which becomes a bad memory, and after three repetitions we look at it with certainty and believe that so much lived experience cannot be wrong. Of course the same applies in reverse to good memories, expectations, experiences, and lived experiences (Figure 2.1).

Ways in which the cycle can be interrupted include creating fictional memories and sending a greeting to the mind with a request to allow this good experience to be perceived as an "always" experience. Memory becomes expectation; what is perceived as an "always" experience is perceived as a "forever" experience. The future in turn consists of expectation – otherwise we would have to say that the future does not exist, because as soon as we get there it has gone – and there is no need to distinguish between "perceived" and "real" expectation. It is exactly the same thing. "Perceived memory" thus leads to a "real expectation".

Jean-Otto Domanski uses the term "reality loop" (inspired by the work of Alexander Hartmann[32]) to describe the same cycle of expectation and memory, albeit oriented less towards the passage of time and more towards physiological experiences and internal images that function as self-fulfilling prophecies. Whereas the

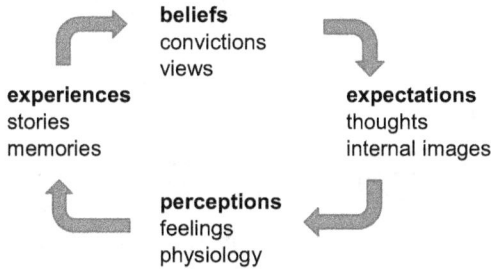

Figure 2.2 Perception, experience, belief, and expectation

"yes set" presupposes a linear development, his model assumes circularity and a circular or spiral consolidation of the experienced "reality".

Domanski describes the cycle as follows:

> Our imagination, our internal images and **expectations** give rise to bodily **perceptions** and feelings and a certain physiology, and thus influence our perception. If this happens a number of times, we call it an **experience** and can tell stories about it. These experiences form a basis for our **convictions** and beliefs, which in turn influence our internal images and perceptions. It is thus that we create our reality.[33]

It is possible to start creating a different reality at any point. Options include ...

• imagining other internal images and films,
• assuming a different posture,[34]
• telling different stories about yourself, or
• developing different convictions and beliefs.

Filter bubble

Anyone who repeatedly accesses certain types of information in search engines, on shopping sites and on social networks, for example by submitting queries on the same topics, will find that similar content is served up to him and different content is increasingly excluded from his attention. The information becomes increasingly similar, increasingly biased and possibly also increasingly radicalised. The phenomenon of self-stabilising information cycles is older than the Internet, however. It typifies the consolidation of traditions and beliefs in religions, ideologies, and national movements. It is representative of processes that build and stabilise roles and identities in a family, in a village, at a workplace, and probably even in a pack of animals. There is accordingly a stabilising function within us that makes us think that our past and future are identical, that we are and always remain the same and that the world also stays the same. If anything in our life remains the same, it does so only because we keep it the same through the constant suggestion that our future is our past ...

Familiarity with cycles of this kind can assist the process of facilitating what is beneficial, for example ...

- a non-anaesthetised operation that is free of pain or involves only a small amount of pain,
- an experience of meaning and value in spite of early and ongoing parental rejection,
- a rapid reduction in acute suicidal tendencies,
- a release from post-traumatic stress,
- fresh courage to face life after a major bereavement,
- a low-symptom or symptom-free withdrawal from an addictive substance.

Much of the above is familiar from hypnosis work. No specific quality or depth of trance is required for this purpose, however, but instead a therapeutic dramaturgy which ...

- deconstructs relevance and plausibility for the problem experience, and
- constructs and stabilises relevance and plausibility for the solution experience.

2.1.3 Separating, linking, and transforming

A "problem" is a discrepancy between how things are and how they should be in the eyes of the individual who perceives the situation as a problem. No situation is a problem in and of itself. It is the observer who decides that, "things are not right here". Whether we regard certain circumstances as a "problem" depends on whether we look at them through a "problem lens". This does not change the fact that certain value judgements mean that it is sometimes easy for us to regard a context as a problem and difficult for us to identify a resource or a solution in it.

A "resource" is everything that can contribute to a solution. Things are not pre-destined to be resources or solutions. A resource becomes a resource based on the judgement of an observer who perceives something useful in it ("that is how it should be"). Instead of talking about "solutions", we can also talk about a solution experience. This makes it clear that it is often more effective to change perspectives than to alter external circumstances if the aim is to achieve a liberating experience.

The general principle is as follows: *the therapist should behave in such a way that problems are separated, solutions are linked and problems are transformed into solutions* (Figure 2.3).[35]

"Separating problems" means: problem-associated topics are differentiated (dissociated, fragmented) until they are not experienced as a burden and they also do not indirectly promote such an experience, namely ...

- within themselves (integrity),
- from each other (diversity),

- from the ego experience (identity),
- from the current experience (reality),
- from the now (present),
- from the duration (reliability),
- from the here (current location),
- and from solution aspects (resources, skills).

Problems can be separated from each other, from something or from the ego experience extremely effectively if they are linked to something else, namely the opposite of the variable from which they are to be separated.

If the therapist wants to separate a problem from the client's ego, he can link it to the "he", "she", or "it" of her body, her mind, or another authority in the third person. If the client says, "I'm suffering," instead of responding with the words, "You're suffering," the therapist is more likely to say, "Your body is suffering," or "Your mind is suffering."

If he wants to separate a problem from the client's experience of reality, he can link problem-associated sentences with "would be" phrases; i.e. instead of agreeing that, "the way things currently are is bad," he will tend to say, "it would be bad if it were to stay like that."

In order to separate the problem from the client's experience of the present, the therapist can choose a verb in the past tense. If a client states, "I often have migraines," the therapist can reflect the sentence back with a slight alteration: "Up until now you've often had migraines." If the therapist perceives a certain amount of confidence in the client already, he can be somewhat bolder: "Up until now you *have* often *had* migraines," or, even more daringly, "Up until now you often *had* migraines," or even, "Up until now you *had* often *had* migraines." He chooses the boldest wording he believes will not trigger a protest (or in other words no internal anti-suggestion).

"Linking solutions" means: things that are connected to resource experiences, skill experiences, and solution experiences are linked (associated, identified) within each other and with each other from the same points of view until they are experienced more and more often as beneficial and conducive.

In turn, solutions can be effectively linked to each other, to the client's ego experience or to something else by separating them from the dissociative wordings of the client (or the therapist).

If the client says, "It would be great if it were to stay like that," the therapist can suggest, "Would it also be OK with you if we said, 'It is great if it stays like that?'"

If the therapist is working in line with the therapeutic modelling method and a client sits down in the space where she had previously described herself as the person for whom things are going well, it might be the case that the client says, "*The person sitting here* feels good, somehow lighter and freer." The therapist can answer, "*You* feel good here, definitely lighter and freer, is that right? How can you tell?" The client typically answers in the first person: "I'm breathing more freely, I have a clear head, I feel like I can see clearly." The outcome of the above is that the experience that has been described is identified with her as an ego experience and largely stabilised.

"Transforming problems into solutions" means transforming a problem experience into a solution experience in small steps or smooth transitions.

This can be achieved in a number of different ways:

- Bodily sensations are transformed into related, less unpleasant feelings, for example pain into a slight itch or a hot or cold feeling, or they are shifted in the client's imagination to other locations in the body.
- Bodily reactions are transformed into emotions, e.g. skin reactions into irritation.
- Emotionally stressful memories or expectations are linked to stories whose protagonists are firstly burdened, but then increasingly liberated.
- Stress-related "beliefs" are repeated and varied in tone (e.g. sung instead of cried) until a shift in meaning is experienced.[36]

Transformation procedures are most frequently used to shape visual imaginings, by gradually converting an initial image into a target image.

2.1.4 Pacing and leading

In the field of hypnotherapy, reference is often made to "pacing and leading", or in other words the need for the therapist to pace the client in her initial experience, which typically means her problem experience, and then to take on the role of leader. Heated debate rages over the question of the extent to which a therapist should "lead" his client or whether he should instead "pace" her. One thing is certain: the client mentions an experience during the conversation that she experiences as a problem and in respect of which she desires change, in the sense of an improvement or solution. She has not succeeded in achieving this change alone, but in principle she regards a path to a better life as conceivable. That's why she's asked a therapist for support. If the therapist merely wanted to pace the client without contributing anything new that might make a valuable difference for her, the client could save herself the time and expense of going to therapy. If he only led her, however, like in the story about the Boy Scout who helps the old woman over the road whether or not she wants to cross, the client would also be no better off (Figure 2.3).

King and ministers

A balance between consequences and pacing is expressed in the following metaphor: "You are the king. I am your minister. Your GP, your psychiatrist, your social worker are also ministers ... A minister contributes his ideas and his skills, but the king decides who advises him and what should ultimately happen."

Gunther Schmidt expresses something similar with his description of a therapist as a "reality waiter" (by way of analogy to a wine waiter). A waiter explains the dishes to the diner, but the latter decides which one is the right choice for him.[37]

Separate problems ...   **Link solutions ...**

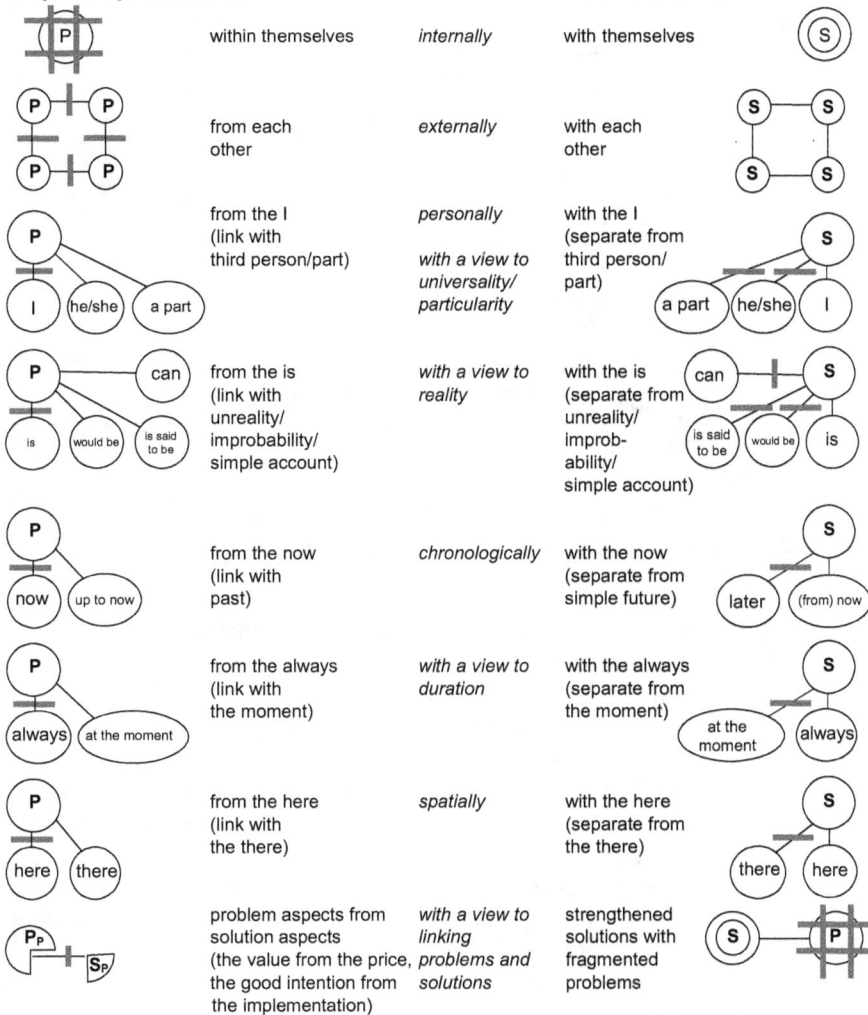

Separate problems		Link solutions
within themselves	*internally*	with themselves
from each other	*externally*	with each other
from the I (link with third person/part)	*personally* / *with a view to universality/ particularity*	with the I (separate from third person/ part)
from the is (link with unreality/ improbability/ simple account)	*with a view to reality*	with the is (separate from unreality/ improb- ability/ simple account)
from the now (link with past)	*chronologically*	with the now (separate from simple future)
from the always (link with the moment)	*with a view to duration*	with the always (separate from the moment)
from the here (link with the there)	*spatially*	with the here (separate from the there)
problem aspects from solution aspects (the value from the price, the good intention from the implementation)	*with a view to linking problems and solutions*	strengthened solutions with fragmented problems

Figure 2.3 Separate problems, link solutions

The therapist's work can involve helping the client to build a bridge from the previous problem experience (P) to a possible solution experience (S), as shown in Figure 2.4.

If I may be permitted to use the phrase, there are two options for reliably making a pig's ear of therapy.

Option 1: the therapist can double down on recognising the gravity of the client's suffering, exploring the problem situation with her and examining every last detail of the problem together. Although the client feels understood and accepted, nothing else changes about her situation (Figure 2.5).

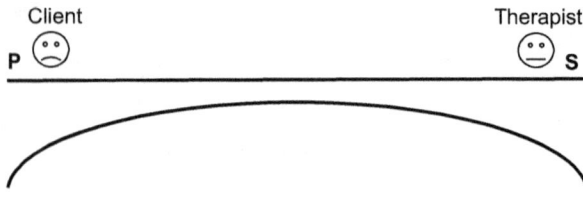

Figure 2.4 Therapy outset

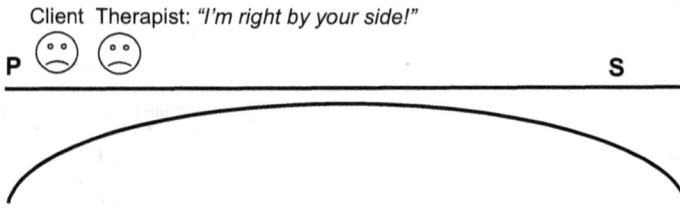

Figure 2.5 Option 1 for therapy failure: Collapsing with the client

Option 2: the therapist can focus on showing the client that happiness and hope are possible, and that good things come by themselves ("Time heals all wounds!") or alternatively that the client merely needs to put in some effort in order to see an improvement. Although the client can see that things are going well for the therapist, the therapist's world is not her world (Figure 2.6).

How might it look if things were different? Instead of using the letters "P" and "S" ("problem" and "solution"), we could also use the letters "P" and "L" in our diagrams to stand for "pacing" and "leading", or in other words using the client's problem experience as a starting point and gradually transitioning to a solution experience in steps that are small but experienced as plausible (Figure 2.7).

Sometimes clients find it easy to search for the path to a better life together with the therapist, and then the therapist can offer positive perspectives relatively early and in concentrated form. The therapist's delight in the fact that the client is solution-oriented should not, however, prompt him to "go to sleep on the job"; instead, he should adapt his (metaphorical) manner and speed of walking to the client's. This is what is meant by "pacing". Sometimes clients find it hard to believe in the possibility of a solution experience. In these cases it can be helpful to take small steps forwards. "The path from hell to heaven is a long one."[38] Sometimes the client cannot or does not want to proceed quickly, and sometimes the gulf between the initial stress and the goal sought is so large that it is a good idea to divide the path into stages, or, to remain with the metaphor of a bridge, to incorporate a few extra piers (Figure 2.8).

In any case, a balance must be struck between the therapist's use of what has been the case to date, or in other words the client's problem experience or initial

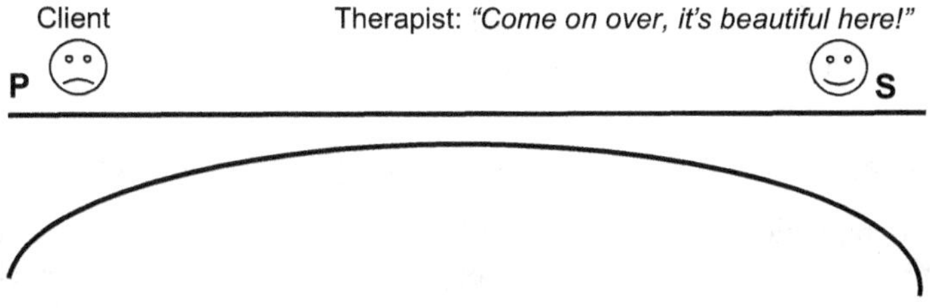

Client   Therapist: *"Come on over, it's beautiful here!"*

Figure 2.6 Option 2 for therapy failure: Letting the client collapse alone

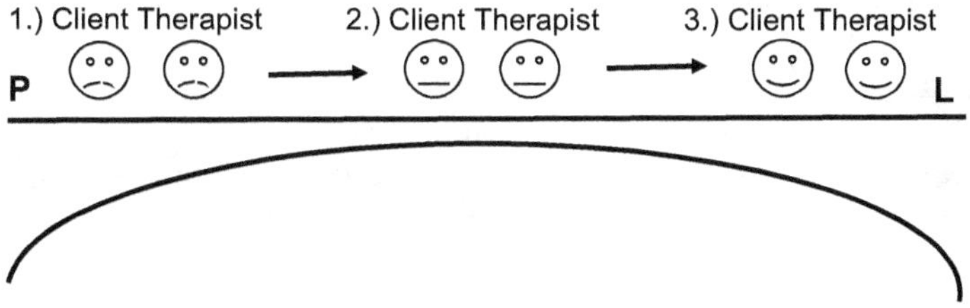

Figure 2.7 Option 1 for therapy success: Moving forward together as quickly as possible

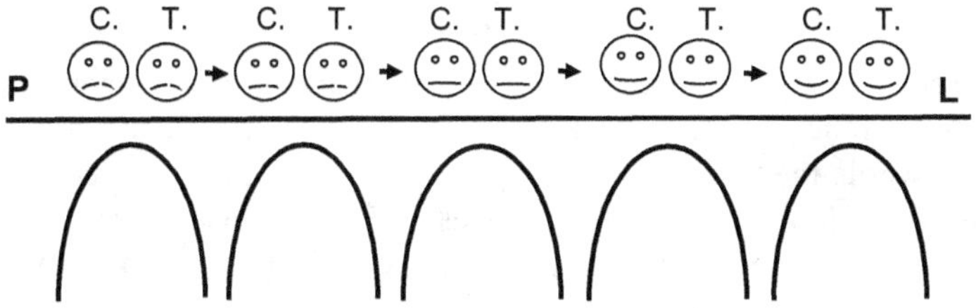

Figure 2.8 Option 2 for therapy success: Moving forward together as slowly as necessary

experience, and approaches which highlight differences from the previous experience that are experienced as helpful and which lead towards a desired target experience.

If pacing alone were on offer, therapists and counsellors would not be able to accomplish the task of showing the client the differences from her previous reality, since the latter would be questioned as a result. If they explain to the client differences that are intended to be productive, however, they may trigger resistance that jeopardises cooperation ... On the one hand, they should support and respect clients' experience in an empathetic and affirmative manner. On the other hand, they should offer change-focused interventions by supporting self-organised searching and finding processes (both conscious and unconscious) in clients that are aimed at a helpful new organisation of patterns.[39]

In this connection, pacing and leading are not primarily two consecutive stages of a process, but instead, and in particular, two complementary sides.

2.2 Assumptions and attitudes from systemic therapy

Systemic therapy did not emerge from systems theory. Over the course of its development it has grappled with systems theory, and to a certain extent warmed to it. In methodological terms, systemic therapy works with the following:

- the valuing and furthering of existing strengths,
- the identification and reproduction of solution strategies that are already successful,
- a wide range of different questioning techniques,
- unfamiliar interpretations of familiar situations,
- the development of vivid visions or clear criteria for what is desired,
- "homework", during which habitual patterns of thinking and behaving can be questioned or new ones tried out.

Finally, the conversations typically leave a lot of room for humour, optimism, and curiosity about life.

2.2.1 Utilisation (use everything!)

As discussed above, utilisation involves using elements of the therapeutic starting point (or in other words the "problem") in order to achieve the target situation (or in other words the "solution"). Elements of this kind may include the client's symptoms, behaviours, values, preferences and aversions, biographical experiences, acquired knowledge, convictions, words, and ideas, but also events in the chronological context of the therapy.

Utilisation is typically associated with Erickson's work, and almost never with systemic work. In reality, almost all traditional systemic techniques are applied forms of utilisation (probably because they can almost all be traced back to Erickson). This includes paradoxical interventions, value-laden connotations, playful work with ambivalences (therapeutic double binds), therapeutic rituals, observation tasks, and the technique of reframing. [40]

If I had to list the top three principles of utilisation, they would probably be the following.

1. Value everything brought to you by the client and the situation! Look for a resource, a skill, and an opportunity in everything!
2. Use everything brought to you by the client and the situation! Look for a contribution to achieving the goals of therapy in everything!
3. Look for the potential good intention of any event, however unfavourable! Expect a desire for safety, belonging, and well-being to be hiding behind everything!

It goes without saying that some of what we are brought by clients initially appears – to them and to us – not worthy of being valued. For example, what about …

- suicidal and self-harming clients?
- clients with a paranoid worldview?
- violent or sexually intimidating clients?
- clients who do not respect us?

The simplest route is to stipulate that some of it is simply valueless.

But the dilemma is that if we do not succeed in seeing clients as absolutely valuable, even with this behaviour and experience, they either will not accept us or will not find a way to accept themselves and others.

On the other hand, if we succeed in finding them (and potentially something about their behaviour) valuable, they might discover that they do not need to replace the elements of their life, but merely to rearrange them so that matters can improve.

We should most definitely avoid trivialising people's suffering by emphasising what is good about the bad things that they have done to themselves or to others, or that they themselves have suffered. Yet the following question remains.

How can we discover what is valuable behind what is harmful so that clients build a positive future on the basis of what exists, which is already working in a dysfunctional manner, instead of searching for something that they are unfamiliar with and incapable of?

The therapist can ask his client:

- Since when has this been present in your life, and what else was happening back then?
- Had you already faced similar challenges beforehand?
- Are you aware of any particular challenges at the start of your life?
- If so, did one of your parents face similar challenges as well?

The therapist can ask himself, and perhaps also his client:

- What purpose might this behaviour and experience have served at the time?
- How might we interpret it as an attempt by the body to relieve the burden?
- What might the body's good intention have been when it created the symptom?

If the therapist still lacks inspiration after working through these questions, he can try the following:

- He can specify when, in which subdomain, or owing to which misunderstanding a good intention might have existed.
- He can take a transgenerational approach, an approach that serves the interests of a larger system or the subfunctions of the body, or an evolutionary approach.

- He can acknowledge both sides of an ambivalence or a conflict of interest.
- He should never assign value to the activity that causes suffering, but can certainly do so to the suffering or misunderstanding that led to it.
- Sometimes it is safer to respect things silently than with words.

What works or does not work is a question of perspective. The therapist can practise recognising what works in what does not work and what does not work in what works:

- What works for one goal might not work for another goal (*OCD, conflict of ambivalence*).
- What works for a group might not work for an individual (*bullying*).
- What works for an individual might not work for a group (*"L'État, c'est moi"*).
- What works for one group might not work for another (*apartheid*).
- What works for one subgroup might not work for the whole (*mafia*).
- What works for the whole might not work for a subgroup (*expropriation*).

The therapist can look at what is working, namely …

- in what is not working! (*Look for the good intention!*),
- between what is not working! (*Look for the exceptions!*),
- next to what is not working! (*Look at other areas of life!*),
- outside what is not working! (*Look at other living beings!*),
- before what is not working! (*Look at what has succeeded in the past!*),
- after what is not working! (*Look at the world of possibilities!*),
- in areas that are allegedly irrelevant! (*Look at trivialities!*).

The therapist can look at everything that works, that is obvious and indisputable for the client, and that is likely to be a "well-beaten track" in the client's mind. He can look at …

- what has worked for a particularly long time or often,
- what is well networked (with many events, people, thoughts),
- what is unusual,
- what is associated with particular skills,
- what is valuable and emotionally charged,
- what is perceptible using the external senses or in the imagination,
- what can be experienced spatially and at the present time.

In order to deconstruct what is not working as a subjective experience, he can relate …

- what works to what does not work, as a priority – or in other words as relevant, plausible, or sensorily or emotionally intense (*"You're very strong-willed!*

Decide for yourself when you want to soil yourself, and write it down in this table."),

- what does not work to itself, paradoxically! (*"Brilliant! A perfect mistake!"* *"The person inside you who says, 'I can't do anything,' shouldn't worry you. She can't do anything, she says so herself."*),
- *one* thing that doesn't work to the *other* thing that doesn't work in order to destabilise one or both of them! (*"It's not right that I've been somewhere you've wanted to visit for your entire life. You can't commit suicide until you've seen the Białowieża National Park. Go there first."*[41]),
- what is not working to what is working in order to destabilise what is not working! (*"Please summon the successful one as a coach for the one who has drunk too much in the evening up until now, and the evening connoisseur for the one who works too hard."*[42] *"Let's agree on the following: for each cigarette that you smoke, you have to donate five euros to the political party you hate the most."*[43]).

How can something like this that does not work have come into being? What might be the good intention behind a behaviour or experience that causes harm and benefits no one? The therapist can …

- talk about intentions such as a striving for safety, belonging, recognition, freedom to act, and freedom from suffering in relation to unsuitable implementation strategies,
- not talk about the good intention of disasters (or an underlying force of fate), but instead about the values on behalf of which we are suffering, for example,
- talk about what is nevertheless to be valued in what is bad, in recognition of the suffering of those affected, out of respect for them and all of humanity.

If, working on this basis, the therapist still dares to remain on the lookout for what can be valued in what appears to be useless and harmful, he has the following option: he can be alert to errors in the system – misunderstandings with the best of intentions, so to speak – when symptoms arise. Misunderstandings of this kind are present in the human organism, not only in parts that appear to us to be solely of the body, but also in those we regard as of the mind. Yet they are also present in families, companies, clubs, official authorities, ethnic communities, and civic societies. The system might have followed a fatal logic that has often proved successful yet is no longer successful in a certain situation (or from then on):

- What feels bad is bad.
- What feels good is good.
- Hope is a precondition for disappointment, and should therefore be avoided.
- Trust is a precondition for abuse, and should therefore be avoided.
- Happiness is a precondition for unhappiness, and should therefore be avoided.
- Combating emotions means regulating emotions.
- If an action has not helped, do more of the same so that it helps.

- If an action has helped, there's no need to do anything else to keep things the same.
- If an action has helped, keep doing it so that things stay the same.
- If an action helped previously, it will also help at a later date.
- If an action did not help previously, it also will not help at a later date.
- What I can't imagine doesn't exist.
- Fear helps against danger.
- The danger is as great as the fear.
- The danger is as small as the fear.
- To be on the safe side, choose the lesser of two challenges!
- To be on the safe side, choose the greater of two challenges!
- Anger helps against powerlessness.
- Talking is thinking out loud and has similar effects.
- Thinking is talking in your head and has similar effects.
- If I only think something, it has no effect on my environment.
- If someone is not told something, it has no effect on him.
- If things happen at the same time, there is a causal relationship between them.
- Once the specific cause has been forgotten, vague justifications are helpful.

Utilisation is an attitude rather than a technique – an attitude of valuing and using everything brought to the therapist by the client, her system, and the current working situation.

2.2.2 What remains the same and what changes: circularity and disrupting patterns

The above list of misunderstandings is also a collection of beliefs that can persist for an arbitrary length of time because they appear to be self-confirming or at any rate are not refuted by anything.

The following argument might be advanced in response to this. "The fact that fear doesn't help against danger – to pick just one example – is something you'd notice as soon as it didn't help." On the other hand, however, someone plagued by anxiety might believe the following: "If I'd been less aware of the danger, my reaction might have been even worse." A belief of this kind can be difficult to refute. To the person plagued by anxiety, trying even more fear next time does not seem like a far-fetched idea, since last time the fear appeared to be justified:

> The symptom develops into a spiral of increasing avoidance and concomitantly growing fear. It is only through avoidance that the fear become autonomous, dysfunctional and chronic. What emerges is a growing fear of fear itself.[44]

One might easily be reminded of the conversation between the little prince and the drunkard who states that he is drinking in order to forget that he is ashamed because he is drinking.[45]

Everything that works similarly or identically over a long period of time is stabilised by control loops and interlocking cycles whose functioning is not apparent to us in most instances. And what escalates is also kept in motion by control loops of this kind ...

We need yet more histamines! (Spirals of escalation)

Perhaps an allergic attack is when the body has noticed that an unusually large amount of histamines are circulating. In my imagination, I can see someone in there calling out: "So many histamines! They must be there for a reason! There must be some impending danger! We need more histamines to face the danger!" Then someone else calls out: "There's even more histamines! The danger must be even greater! We need yet more histamines!"

There can be no question about the fact that conflicts between partners, rival groups, or nations work similarly. When a couple argues, for example, it is to be expected that the first partner's response to the second's action is the action to which the second responds. Both partners believe that they are responding to the other's aggressive impulses and protecting themselves by means of behaviours that are deemed aggressive by the other and that prompt them to protect themselves by means of behaviours deemed aggressive by the other, and on and on.

If a client responds to a challenging situation that persists for a long time with destructive dream images or internal dialogues, it is to be expected that her dreams are not merely the result of this situation, but also a sustaining force for it.[46]

Every recurring event that appears to be the consequence of another recurring event in a stable system may at the same time be its cause.

Recurring structures are parts of a pattern into which the problem experience is so embedded that it stabilises itself. With a view to understanding how the experienced problem can be transformed, it is a good idea to describe patterns of action, interaction, and interpretation:

- that can be used as a model to explain the problem,
- that generate the problem (and that might maintain it, speaking circularly),
- that give rise to the problem as an outcome,
- that give rise to everything and therefore also the problem (space, time, causality, perception, identity).

Convictions that cause suffering, either directly or indirectly, can also be destabilised through questions or over-stabilised through intensification – or both at the same time![47]

Patterns of behaviour and experience can be identified in many areas. Provided that we do not "cling" to our own models and believe that we are describing a reality without alternatives, it is a good idea to practise developing hypotheses for patterns of this kind in a playful manner, extrapolating from what is visible, known, and obvious to the underlying life experiences in the process!

We can explore the following, for example:

- memory styles, current perception and interpretation, expectation styles (*interpretations of reality*),
- verbal communication structures (*grammar, metaphors*),
- verbal and communicative interaction structures (*hierarchies, reciprocally reinforcing messages, misunderstandings, agreements*),
- non-verbal visible communication (*physical behaviour, clothing etc.*),
- non-verbal audible communication (*tone of voice, volume, clearing one's throat etc.*),
- what is felt physically and emotionally by clients or by the therapist himself,
- behavioural habits, rituals, conditioned reactions,
- corporate, cultural, and family traditions,
- professional and family experiences, skills that can be deduced on this basis,
- likes (*preferences*) and dislikes (*aversions*),
- convictions (*opinions, beliefs, and values*),
- symptoms and the prerequisites and consequences that can be deduced on this basis.

Using systemic questions[48] and working together with clients, the therapist can develop ideas about the patterns that serve as a basis for their interpretation and shaping of their lives, and what might be more expedient instead of the previous behaviour and experience.

The systemic techniques to be mentioned in this connection include **reframing**. This term means that the therapist takes the information brought to him by the client and reflects it back to the client from a new perspective, resulting in an explicit or implicit reassessment of the situation.[49]

In the following example, the therapeutic intervention refers to the original situation described by the couple (*situational reframing*).

So much love

A couple came to therapy and complained that they were no longer communicating well and were often ending up in conflict with each other. The woman explained that whenever her husband was not at work, he would always disappear off to the construction site where their new house was going to be built. She said that although she understood the amount of time involved in building a house, it seemed to her like he was no longer present in her life at all. She felt abandoned, like a single parent who was raising the children without any help. As she saw it, he never had any time for her or the children, and she wasn't really sure any more why they'd got married. The husband said that his wife simply could not grasp the sheer effort involved in building a house for a family. He felt that she did nothing but criticise him, and that she never showed any appreciation for his contribution to the family.

I explained to both of them that I was amazed by the depth of their love. I said that it was quite obvious to me that the woman was aware that construction delays might result in extra expense and complications, but that closeness with her husband and being together as a family were what mattered most to her. I went on to say that the husband could undoubtedly imagine much nicer ways to spend his evenings and all of his weekends than hanging around on a building site; it would certainly be much more pleasant for him as well to spend them sitting at home on the sofa, chatting with his wife, and playing with his children, but his love for his wife and children meant that he was willing to make this sacrifice. "I've never thought about it like that," said the wife, and the husband agreed that this was a helpful perspective.

Paradigmatic reframing is also possible. The therapist can continue as follows:

Red roses

I once knew a woman who confessed the following to me. "My husband has bought red roses for me throughout our entire marriage. I've never told him that I find creamy white roses much nicer. I've always thought that if he really loved me, he'd notice all on his own."[50] That's a shame, isn't it? I'm delighted that you've come to see me. By taking this time to say exactly what you want, you're giving each other the opportunity to express your love for each other in such a way that the message is also heard and understood!

It is also possible to use *metaphorical reframings*. For example, the therapist can continue as follows:

Packages of love

If you don't receive any love, there are several reasons why that might be the case. Perhaps the packages of love were sent off properly and arrive safely, but you're currently away on holiday. The post office keeps packages that have not been delivered for a week, but then returns them to the sender. Perhaps the packages of love were sent off properly but don't arrive. It might be that the address is illegible, or that something's wrong with the postage. Maybe the package was parcelled up but never got sent. Or maybe there were problems in the shipping department. I'd only start considering the possibility that there might be no love left in stock as an absolute last resort – and when I see you in front of me, I really don't think that's the case.

Most systemic interventions such as paradoxical interventions, rituals, or observation tasks have their roots in the concept of utilisation. Reference should be made to the relevant literature for a more detailed description of this concept.[51]

2.2.3 Resources, contexts, relationships, futures, goals, and solutions

Hypnosystemic therapy takes the fundamental attitudes of systemic therapy as a reference point for values and actions and expands these attitudes to include a number of fresh perspectives. Its focus is correspondingly also on resources, contexts, relationships, potential futures, goals, and solutions; the understanding of these focal points merely differs sometimes from the traditional systemic approach.

Resource orientation means the following: generally speaking, the opportunities and possibilities available to individuals come to the fore. The special abilities of the recipient of counselling (a person or a group and its members) are highlighted and strengthened. The focus is not placed on shortcomings. Personal "weaknesses" are regarded as subjective perceptions that might furthermore be temporary in nature, since they depend to a large extent on the perspectives and behaviours of the group members or the individual's self-perception, which can change. Instead of "resources", Gunther Schmidt often talks about the "skills" of an individual or a system,[52] thereby valuing the creative power of the system and its members.

In *hypnosystemic* work, it is expected that the client's unconscious and the system surrounding her will hold enormous potential in terms of unknown resources. Instances in the client's body can stimulate solutions that the client's conscious would not initially view as realistic. Every goal that is set is therefore subject to the proviso that outcomes surpassing those sought at the start are also regarded as achievable in principle, and will be realised wherever possible.

Context and relationship orientation means the following: instead of assigning personal traits to individuals, we talk about the behaviour they demonstrate and the contexts in which this occurs. Even an involuntary experience is regarded not as an immutable characteristic of an individual; instead, it is viewed contextually as an expression of his current relationship with himself and his environment. The perspectives and behaviours of the individuals in a network of relationships are therefore examined in terms of their interactions. The question subject to consideration and testing is as follows: which new ways of relating to one another, together with their impacts, might lead to increased satisfaction levels, ideally among everyone involved?

The responsibility of individuals and the particular stresses they face are not viewed in isolation, but interpreted as the expression of relationships within the social system.

Causalities in networks of relationships tend to be viewed in a circular rather than in a linear sense, or in other words in terms of reciprocal and reticular (field-like) influences.

In *hypnosystemic* work, the relationships between the sides (parts, options) of the personality (for example, the internal accuser and the internal accused) are constructed and treated like relationships between physical people. The possibility of mediation talks between the internal parties to the conflict can be offered. Alternatively, these sides can be treated like mythical creatures or animated figures that can be transformed into any imaginable shape, in order to generate plausible solutions following the logic of these genres that can be experienced by clients as relevant to their own action and experience.

Parallel contexts are often constructed for the purpose of identifying solutions; for example, in a story with a protagonist whose problem has similarities with the client's story or by means of a problem landscape that is transformed into a solution landscape.[53]

Future orientation means the following: in traditional systemic counselling, the focus of attention tends not to be on the past, since the past cannot be altered.

In *hypnosystemic* work, the past is viewed as a memory in the present (including bodily reactions and emotions, interpreted as physiological memories) and as mutable. Examining memories is interpreted as pacing, on the basis of which reactions that previously caused suffering can be altered (leading).

Goal and solution orientation means the following: opportunities for change that benefit from the broadest possible consensus between the participants are typically sought. What matters is searching for achievable goals and solutions to achieve a greater level of satisfaction among those involved, as well as starting the implementation of changes in reciprocal perception and behaviour. "Goal orientation" can also be described as "mission orientation"; the counsellor initially identifies the mission which the client has assigned him to support the achievement of her goals, and then pursues this mission consistently until the interlocutors conclude that the goal that was set has been achieved or that the client has altered her goal.

Differences do, however, exist between the definition of goals from a traditional systemic perspective and a hypnosystemic perspective.

From the traditional systemic perspective, goals should be …

… *formulated positively*, or in other words: "I want …" instead of "I don't want …".

In *hypnosystemic* work, we can furthermore dissociate everything that is undesirable for the client from her ego experience (e.g. visualise and externalise stresses) until nothing else worries her. She will then typically be able to formulate what she needs in precise and positive terms. Alternatively, she can test out how it feels to identify more and more with the approximate opposite of the problem experience or with a physiology that is incompatible with it. If the client wants to "get rid of this awful anxiety," we can place in the room the person who she is when she experiences "confidence", "satisfaction", and "curiosity," or if she "sits there and relaxes", "breathes calmly", and "listens with interest". We can let her experience who she is as this person, and stabilise this condition with her if it proves successful from the client's perspective.

… *formulated in concrete terms*, or in other words as a description of a perceptible behaviour.

In *hypnosystemic* work, we do not need to know what it means for the client to be "happy again at last". Her unconscious knows it, and that is enough. If we take out of the world of possibilities and place in the room the person, "who you are when you are happy again at last", and ask the client to describe her posture, facial expression, voice etc., she will do just that, and if we ask her to sit down over there and to experience how it is to be this person, she will, generally speaking, also experience just this.

… *achievable*, so that their implementation is 100% within the client's control.

In *hypnosystemic* work, we can also work with "the image of your partner from your head". We can find out how the internally experienced relationship between the client and her family members can change in a beneficial way. Then we can stabilise the modified internal image, combined with the associated physiology and emotionality, and allow it to radiate onto the real relationships. It is likely that the family members will behave differently towards the client because she involuntarily sees and treats them differently.

Every individual's experience of identity in a social structure is the result of how she is viewed by each of the others in the structure, provided that she does not raise any objections to this point of view. If the client sees her family members in a helpfully different manner, the identities assigned to her by herself and others change, and therefore also the framework of roles in the system.

... *realistic*, so that achievement of the goal is possible and likely.

In *hypnosystemic* work, a distinction is made between the creative possibilities of conscious experience and those of the unconscious. Something that is not consciously achievable by the client might very well be achievable by her unconscious, with which we are communicating. If we do not know whether her unconscious can achieve a goal (for example healing her of a serious illness), we can "pretend that it works" and find out together with her the extent to which her unconscious can realise her goals.

... *neither too small nor too big*, so that the goal is attractive.

In *hypnosystemic* work, small goals can serve as a good basis for pacing the client's hopes (which may still be faint), and big goals can serve as a good basis for leading (in terms of providing a helpful overall focus of attention). Behind every horizon is another horizon, and behind even the best goals that can be imagined at present may be other goals. If we suppose that the most important thing about a goal is that it allows needs to be met, big goals can potentially also be achieved in a short space of time in a dream-like fashion by altering the strategy for implementing these needs.

... *measurable*, so that outcomes can be monitored.

In *hypnosystemic* work, it is often sufficient for the imagined goal to be perceptible to the inner eye and ear, to bodily sensation and to the world of emotions, and for this experience, free from the influence of any objections by internal and external authorities, to become part of the client in the long term. The measurable part of the goals that have been set will then be achieved autonomously by the client's body.

2.2.4 Asking good questions

Good questions are part of the basic toolbox of systemic therapy.[54] It goes without saying that asking questions allows the therapist to gain information, but what matters more is the knowledge that can be gained by the client while searching for the right answer. The questions that are really effective are not those that can be answered by the client without any real thought, but those that trigger an internal search.[55]

Questions are furthermore used to introduce new ideas in systemic and hypnosystemic work. Precisely because questions do not appear to make any assertions, they have enormous suggestive potential (whether deliberately or not). By focusing attention on particular points of view they block out other possible perspectives, and since attention is typically directed at answering the main thrust of the questions, most of their implications are accepted without discussion, and added to the repertoire of automatic thought in the process. Even if the therapist attempts to ask a question neutrally, the precise wording has such an enormous impact on the outcome that key aspects of the answer can often be predicted.[56]

I'd like to share a few observations to illustrate this point.

If I ask seminar participants after we've been working for 90 minutes, "Would you guys like a 15-minute break?" the participants are highly likely to answer "Yes". No thought is given to the option of requesting a 20-minute break, because they were not asked about it. If I ask: "Would you guys like a 20-minute break?" a 20-minute break will be agreed.

If I ask: "Would you guys like to break for 15 or 20 minutes?" a 20-minute break will be chosen. If two equivalent options are offered, the second is almost always chosen.

If I offer the choice of breaking for "20, 25, or 30 minutes", participants will opt for a 25-minute break. If three equivalent options are offered, the middle one is almost always chosen.

If I suggest breaking for "15, 20, 25, or 30 minutes", participants will normally opt for a 25-minute break. If there are four equivalent options, people opt for the third; this is a combination of the two rules (the middle of three equivalent options will be chosen, and the last of two equivalent options will be chosen).

If I make my voice sound subtly more pleasant or interesting when describing the first of two options than when describing the second, the first will be chosen. Differences in intonation take precedence over the order in which options are presented. The same applies if I lend greater significance to the option that is normally inferior through facial expressions or gestures, pauses in speech or a louder voice.

If I state in advance that people almost always choose the second of three equivalent options, the third will almost always be chosen. The middle option has been discredited, and so the situation is set up in such a way that only the first and last options are valid choices.

If I ask, "How long a break would you like?" I have to wait a very long time for a reply. In the end someone will normally suggest breaking for 15 or 30 minutes, depending on how long the previous breaks have normally been.

Regardless of what is being suggested, the outcome can be predicted with a very high level of probability. Rules like the ones described above can be applied to questions about any other topic and to questions worded in any format. As soon as a speaker knows which type of questions ordinarily provoke which answers, he can no longer ask anything without engaging in manipulation. The simplest response that answers the question correctly in formal terms will be the response that is given. This is more or less always the case unless the answer is incompatible with the answerer's interests. It is harder to predict the answers to questions relating to less trivial topics, because the answerer's interests are often not known to the questioner.

Questions always focus attention – asking neutral questions is quite simply impossible

It is therefore all the more important for therapists to keep in mind where their questions are focusing their clients' attention; do they guide clients towards an expansion of their options for thinking and acting, or towards a narrowing of these latter? Do they steer clients towards a more intensive focus on shortcomings and problems, or towards a focus on skills and solutions? Do they direct clients' focus towards rigidity or flexibility, fears or hopes, powerlessness or relief?

Certain types of systemic questions have become more widely known, and are described below.

CIRCULAR QUESTION

"If I were to ask your daughter what makes your husband drink, what do you think she would say?"

SCALING QUESTION

"Imagine a scale that runs from zero to ten, where zero means that you'd like to stop studying right away and ten that you'd definitely like to keep on studying, whereabouts on this scale are you? Would you rather have a higher or lower value on the scale?"

EITHER/OR QUESTION

"Would you rather see the ADHD which the paediatrician has diagnosed in your son, if that is what it is, as having been present from his birth or acquired at some later point in time?"

HYPOTHETICAL QUESTION

"Supposing that therapists didn't exist, what would you be doing instead of being here?"

EXCEPTION QUESTION

"At what times do you not observe the problem?"

MIRACLE QUESTION

"If a fairy godmother were to come along tonight and conjure away your problem, and you didn't realise what had happened at first because you were asleep, when and how would you notice it tomorrow?"

From a therapeutic perspective, what clients answer to these questions is often less important than the fact that engaging with them opens up fresh perspectives and thus fresh options for ways in which to think and act.[57]

In *hypnosystemic* therapy, questions of this kind can be used with great effect to stimulate the client's unconscious to search for new ideas and perspectives that have not yet been discovered through conscious thought.

There are also a number of other questions that have proven very successful, as explained below.

QUESTION ABOUT WHERE THE CLIENT THINKS THE PROBLEM MIGHT HAVE ORIGINATED

It is astonishingly often the case that clients spend a long time *not* telling the therapist what they believe might be causing the problem, and it is astonishingly often the case that therapists do not ask them to do so (probably because they think that clients will volunteer this information of their own accord), and it is astonishingly often the case that any course of therapy would be much shorter if the therapist were to ask:

"What do *you* think the origin of the problem might be?"

QUESTION ABOUT THE BEST POSSIBLE OUTCOME OF THE SESSION

"Supposing that this session were to deliver outcomes that were the best possible – or even better – from the point of view of where we are right now, what will you experience afterwards that is different to before?"

One of the aims pursued with this question is preparing the client for an excellent outcome of the therapy. The phrase "from the point of view of where we are right now", like the words "or even better", implies that even better outcomes will be possible from a later point of view. Without these words, we might generate an expectation that once the specified outcome has been achieved, nothing further is possible, and perhaps even that the outcome cannot be achieved in full, because perfection is never or almost never achieved.

The use of the word "supposing" and a verb in the subjunctive mood at the start of the sentence ensures that the client does not discuss the matter or start to question whether these best possible outcomes are actually achievable. In this way any nascent hopes are smuggled unobtrusively past the gatekeeper responsible for reality checks, or more accurately "checks of presumed realities"; in actuality, the goals that are perceived as overly ambitious have very often been met or exceeded by the end of the session. Continuing the sentence in the indicative rather than the subjunctive ("what will you experience" rather than "what would you experience") ensures that what is initially introduced as a simple assumption is now treated as an achievable reality, in order to pave the way for a good expectation to turn into a good experience.

In the therapeutic context, "different" means "better", because the aim of therapy is for something to be different, or in other words better. It is more advantageous to use the word "different" rather than "better", however, because if things that will become "better" are identified, the client's sceptical guardian might repeatedly censor ideas and express concerns in order to prevent the client from nourishing hopes that will only end in disappointment and might then cause pain. This is not what is wanted in therapy; if a positive expectation is reduced, the potential for future positive experiences is always reduced at the same time.

QUESTION ABOUT POTENTIAL TRIGGER EVENTS

"Since when have you felt like that? And what else was happening at the time?"

The dual question is aimed at identifying possible trigger events for physical, mental or social symptoms. This follows the rule of defocusing and refocusing[58] and helps to decouple symptoms and stressful experiences from the current trigger situations by linking them again with the original triggers (which have perhaps already consciously been forgotten).

In order to identify chains of potential traumas and at the same time also larger correlations between stressful events, we can continue to ask:

"When was the first time you felt or behaved like that, or an early situation when it happened?"

"Had you ever known anything similar to happen beforehand?"

"Does the behaviour of the individual involved in this conflict situation remind you of the behaviour of anyone else from an earlier time?"

"Was there anything special in the first few years of your life that might perhaps have meant that situations of this kind are such a challenge for you?"

"Have you ever known one of your parents to display a behaviour like this or to have an experience like this?"

"How long do you think this has been present in your family?"

QUESTION ABOUT PERMISSION TO INTERRUPT

It is often a good idea to ask for permission to interrupt at the start of a session:

"Forgive me if I interrupt you. It won't be that I'm being rude or that I'm bored by what you're saying. I'd love to spend a long time listening to exactly what you have to say. It's just that I'd like permission to interrupt you if I think that we might make faster progress by heading off in a different direction – is that OK?"

Clients will typically respond in the affirmative to a question of this kind, and afterwards the therapist can hopefully interrupt the conversation without seeming impolite whenever necessary if that helps to take it in a new direction.

It is a good idea to offer the client a great deal that can facilitate helpful change so that towards the end of the session she experiences that lots has changed for the better and there is hope of improvement. In the interest of saving time, it is not a good idea to allow her to talk about her problem for a long time at the start.[59]

Building trust is important, but that does not depend specifically on how long the therapist listens to the client at the start of the session, and instead on the client experiencing the therapist's empathic approach as authentic.

QUESTION ABOUT THE NEW GOAL

"Supposing that you'd been feeling the way you're feeling now for years, and we can take that as a given, and so you'd have come here today already feeling like that, and supposing our session were now to begin and I'd ask you, 'What is your problem?', what would you say to me then?"

"If you ask your mind to give these perspectives that are now good for you an 'always' feeling, and if your mind does that, and we now take another look at where we are, what is the goal now?"

These questions perform several different functions. They firstly provide the therapist and client with information on which goals have maybe already been achieved and do not need to be worked on any further, and they secondly presume that what has been achieved for now has already been achieved permanently.

The first question uses the structure that has already been explained, with "supposing" and a "would be" structure followed by an "is" structure. No doubts arise in the client's mind, initially because only a mental game is offered, but also later, during the discreet transformation from assumptions to experienced realities, because the mental game has already been accepted. The client does not carry out a further reality check. The question therefore stabilises the client's belief that the outcome of therapy is permanent.

The second question incorporates a "greeting to the mind",[60] which ensures that what has previously been achieved by the client is treated as having been permanently achieved. Since the request is addressed not to the client ("you"), but to an authority in the third person ("your mind"), it is implemented by involuntary authorities and thus removed from the world of objections. In the unlikely event that the client still wants to express doubts in this respect, the sentence leads to a question that is dealt with primarily at the level of conscious thought, because questions insist on answers and because the question concludes the sentence. The implications of the start of the sentence are therefore no longer worked on consciously and – precisely because no objection is raised – are accepted by the unconscious.

QUESTION ABOUT THE INTEGRATION OF RESOURCE EXPERIENCES

"Now you've had this experience, if you think again about the initial situation, what is now different?"

"On the basis of these images and this altered attitude towards life, can you talk to me again about the situation back then and go into more detail?"

The questions link the physiology of the resource experience with the internal film of the previous problem experience.

The first question elicits verbal feedback from the client about how she would feel if the problem situation were to take place now. Experience has shown that the client's feedback paints a very realistic picture of the outcome.

The second question is geared towards non-verbal feedback; while the client is talking about the situation, the therapist determines how stressful or straightforward the simulated situation is for the client now, based on the intensity of audible stress signals (hesitation, stuttering, clearing the throat, a croaky or nasal voice, sobs, a jangling voice etc.).

Both questions invite the client to allow the internal images of remembered or expected problem situations to pass by her again, this time with the emotions and bodily reactions of the established resource experience.

It would be a good idea for a whole network of resources to have been created beforehand (in line with the rule that we should "link solutions") and for the problem experience to have been fragmented into many sub-aspects that are diminished in relevance and plausibility and differ from each other (in line with the rule that we should "separate problems"). Stresses that are experienced as diminished are linked to physical and mental resources that are experienced as enhanced, by way of a "resource vaccination". A "vaccine reaction" is often also seen; even if clients felt completely content beforehand, after this question they often no longer feel quite so good. We have ultimately co-triggered their memories that have been stressful to date, and that are still not their favourite memories. We can continue to ask questions, as described below.

QUESTION ABOUT THE PROGRESS OF THERAPY

"Supposing I'd asked you at the start of the session to think about this situation, would it have been just as unpleasant, or more or less unpleasant?"

The answer is normally that it would have been significantly more unpleasant to imagine the situation before the therapeutic interventions. This ensures that the client no longer focuses on the idea that "the problem is still there, in spite of going to therapy", but instead on the idea that "the problem has lessened enormously as a result of therapy".

Questions generate new information in the therapist's head and the client's head. What is more, they often change the entire focus of the client's attention, her approach to the situation perceived as problematic and the significance she assigns to the previous problem.

2.3 Assumptions and attitudes from psychodrama, constellation work, and parts work

Hypnosystemic work makes liberal use of phenomena that are well known from constellation work, parts concepts, and psychodrama. To name but a few examples, this includes the skills of ...

• viewing aspects of an experience in personified form before the inner eye,

- experiencing oneself as "many",
- putting oneself into another's place in a highly realistic manner,
- experiencing oneself as a particular person even though that may not (yet) be the case,
- experiencing at a bodily level possible ways of living,
- retaining for the benefit of real experience the physiology of an imagined experience.

The techniques listed above fall under the heading of therapeutic modelling.[61] Personified options rather than "parts" are used for the work. The externalised persons do not represent immutable and undetachable components of the client, but rather opportunities for self-experience which her unconscious can choose again (reassociate), remove (permanently dissociate), or reshape (transform).

Viewing burdensome aspects of an experience as "parts" would imply a relatively strong association and identification with the problem experience and problem behaviour. Clients might believe that "parts of the personality" are something that one cannot or should not lose, like "parts of the body". By way of contrast, the aim of therapy is for the client to distinguish between herself and the problem experience and to find ways to live her life without the stress that has previously resulted from the lack of any such distinction.

If we interpret these dissociated forms of clients' experience as "possibilities of their experience", or as the "people they might be" (but do not have to be), we support the idea that change is possible.

Since this way of working differs somewhat from other approaches that visualise imagined persons ("parts" or similar), I'd like to provide several examples that illustrate the possible applications in a therapeutic context.

2.3.1 Inside and outside

We can confront family members and other important people in our lives even if they are not currently in the same room as us, because we carry around with us internal images and films of them! We experience these films as memories, expectations, fantasies (how it might have been or how it could be), or as a mixture of all three. Everything we see, hear, and feel during this process in our imagination is experienced highly realistically, with all of the emotions and all of the physiological reactions. After all, the people who shape our lives are usually not even in our physical vicinity when we argue with them. Even if we hardly ever see them in real life or if they have already died, they continue to take up prime real estate in our heads.

Taking her father out of her head

"I don't want our work to focus on my father. He ruins everything for me," said a woman in therapy. "I don't want our work to focus on your father either,"

I answered. "I don't care about your father. And your father isn't here. You're here. You're the one I'm working with. But what concerns me is that even though your physical father isn't here, your internal image of your father is bossing you around and torturing you. I'd like the father in your head to stop doing that so that you can get some peace. Can we work on that?" "Yes," said the woman. "Then let's try taking the image of your father out of your head. Out of your head and over there!" I pointed to the opposite corner of the room. "Look at him standing over there! How does that feel, now that he's over there and out of your head, and you're over here?" "Much better," said the woman. She was breathing deeply and freely.

There are two reasons why the woman experienced this intervention as liberating. Firstly, it is advantageous to be able to make a distinction between the physical original of an individual and our internal image of him. Secondly, by removing the image of the father out of the woman, we increased the distance between her and her father. This follows the rule that we should "separate problems". It's not about viewing the father as a "problem per se". The woman associates him with the problem in the current context, and hence it is a good idea to make a distinction between her Internal image of her father on the one hand and her ego experience and her here-and-now experience on the other. If the therapist had said, "Let's summon your father into the room with us!" and had assigned to him the same space now occupied by the father removed from the woman's head, her response would probably have been coloured by stress rather than relief. The rule is that we should "link solutions", and not that we should link problems.

The heavenly university of love and wisdom

Sooner or later the day will come when your father has passed away. I can imagine him there on the other side, meeting Jesus and Buddha and all the other loving, wise, holy people, Hildegard von Bingen, Theresa von Avila, and many others who are less well known. They force him to come face to face with the damage he's done, and they don't let him look away. But they also ask: "What must he have suffered before he became someone who would do to his daughter something that no father should ever do to his daughter?" He continues to attend this heavenly university of love and wisdom until he is mature, redeemed and enlightened. Regardless of whether it takes ten years or one hundred years or one thousand years – they have all the time in the world over there. "If the redeemed and enlightened version of your father then returns and stands in front of you here, how does he now look at you?" "He looks as though he's saying, 'I'm sorry!' He looks as though he wants to ask something. And I feel sorry for him somehow."

"What does he say to you? ... Do you think that if he comes back such a changed man, he can feel regret? How does he express it? ... And once he has made even more progress, can he at some point also say to you that you're a fantastic daughter? ... If he spent even longer there, can he perhaps also tell you at some point that he's proud of you? ... How does he look while he's saying that? How does his face look, what is his posture like? ... How do you feel when you hear that?"

Once again, we are "separating problems"; we have manoeuvred the father out of the woman's head and into somewhere beyond the known external world. He is doubly dissociated into the world beyond this one, from which he can no longer interact physically. After that comes the phase of "transforming problems into solutions". The problem father is transformed into a solution father with narrative plausibility. As a solution father, however, he is subject to the rule that we should "link solutions". This means that he can return to the room, and although this time he is summoned from outside and placed in the room, the woman makes no protest. Instead, there are clear indications that her relationship with the father from her head has improved.

Turning once again to the concept of "linking solutions", we can use a yes set to take further the idea of who the client's father is in terms of his potential, after imagining him free from everything he made use of to humiliate himself and others. The process is only summarised here, and will need to be tailored to each client, depending at all times on what is suitable, possible and appropriate for the individual.

A type of purgatory can also be incorporated, where the father experiences a painful process of purification by having to look at what he did without being able to escape. This acknowledges the fact that the client's suffering is serious and must not be trivialised. The image then incorporates pacing for the client's anger, but at the same time avoids the idea of "an eye for an eye". Instead, the question that is raised is whether the client desires atonement, to what extent and in what manner. Experience shows that most people do not need atonement if they experience that their suffering is seen, recognised, and acknowledged as serious and unwarranted, if possible by the individual who inflicted it on them. This rarely happens in the real world; in the first place, however, it is also extremely helpful if a therapist, a pastor, a judge, or another authority figure can recognise this suffering, and in the second place it is possible for the image of the person who inflicted the suffering to pass through such a transformation. In some cases it is also permissible for this transformation to be carried out with a mixture of seriousness and humour.

The heavenly soul cleansing

We can agree that people who were the cause of such suffering must be scrubbed clean after their death with sponges and brushes, in a "heavenly soul cleansing". We touch on the idea that the dirt built up not only as a result of what they did and did not do, but also as a result of what they themselves suffered. We think together about how the bath of souls would need to be designed, which cleaning agents would be used, whether the souls would be washed by previously deceased family members, or whether the job would be performed by servants working in the hereafter (angels or devils?), or whether they would need to clean themselves, and of course other questions such as how they would look and what clothes they would be wearing after leaving the bath once they had been cleaned.

The cartoon-like image and the humorous nature of this approach allow a delicate balance to be struck between potential needs for revenge (pacing of anger) and the desire for the suffering to be seen and recognised on the one hand, and the need to belong on the other (pacing of the desire for acceptance). Once a healthy balance of this kind has been achieved, the client may develop an attitude of inner reconciliation, which should never be demanded, but can nevertheless be healing.

Clients have often said something along the lines of the following in the session following such an intervention:

"I phoned my mother. My father joined in with our conversation. It was the first time we'd had a good chat for a long time, or perhaps even the first time ever." "It's strange – I met up with my father. He's changed. He's become much kinder."

The physical people around us become imagined people inside us. In turn, we can make the people inside us imagined people whom we see around us. How the imagined people treat us determines how we treat them and how we treat ourselves. And how we treat the imagined people around us is how we treat the physical people for whom these imagined people stand. And how we treat the physical people around us determines how they treat us.

If we turn the imagined people who cause us stress and who are *inside us* into people *around us,* our stress is relieved. If we transform the imagined people around us who *cause us stress,* in a manner that is experienced as plausible, into people who are *relieved of stress* and *relieve our stress,* our stress is relieved yet further. If we succeed in building a helpful new relationship with the *imagined* people around us, our relationship with the relevant *physical* people will also change in a helpful manner.

At the start of the conversation, the therapist made a distinction between the "physical father" and "the father in your head". This is true to the motto of "separating problems". The problem father is divided up into the physical original and the copy in the client's head. When the solution father returns from heaven after ten years or one hundred years or one thousand years, the therapist has deliberately forgotten this distinction. The client has also forgotten the distinction, to the extent that she treats the physical father a little like the imagined father who has returned from heaven, and he automatically responds in kind.

The distinction between the physical and the imagined father has a perceived plausibility. After all, the people in our head are not the people who they know themselves to be. On the other hand, what do we ever really know about other people except for the image that we have of them in our head? Even if someone is standing right in front of me, I only have the image of him in my head, and never the actual person. There might be a difference between the world around us and the world inside us, but there is no difference as far as our mind and our behaviour are concerned. To put it more precisely, the distinction between inside and outside only exists if we distinguish between them. The therapist has the option of making this distinction whenever it is beneficial to the work ("separating problems") or not making it when *this* is beneficial to the work ("linking solutions").

2.3.2 "I" as many

We can not only externalise our images of certain people, but also personify and externalise any other experiences, for example …

- symptoms of illness and pain,
- bodily reactions that indicate stress (*frowning, clearing one's throat*),
- behaviour and behavioural impulses (*the person who is suicidal, cuts himself, or overeats*),
- emotions such as sadness, fear, or anger,
- reactions of paralysis and numbness (*confusion, emptiness, depression*),
- figures who raise objections to the effectiveness of therapy (*scepticism*),
- the child who the client was when something bad happened (*trauma*).

In line with the principle of "separating problems", problem-associated experiences are personified and dissociated out of the client, and projected onto a place in the room. The burden felt by the client (or the adverse impact which the phenomenon has on the therapeutic work) diminishes at the moment when the client …

- imagines a person of this kind leaving her body,
- assigns to this person a specific place where she sees her from then on,
- describes this person's appearance, voice etc.,
- notices and describes her altered physiology (including emotions).

It is not necessary to speculate about these alterations in experience, since they can typically be identified directly from changes in the client's facial expressions, gestures, breathing, circulation, and movements.

Instead of dissociating individual aspects of stress from the "I", it is also possible to dissociate two or more sides of an ambivalence from the "I" and from each other. I suggested the following to a Syrian refugee called Hassan (not his real name), who was finding it hard to deal with the fact that he didn't know whether his younger brother was still alive or had died in the turmoil of the civil war.

The three Hassans

"Imagine that the Hassan who believes that your younger brother is dead could step out of you and stand opposite you. Look at him standing there, desperately sad and perhaps even crying, with drooping shoulders. Or perhaps he's not even standing, but crouching down or cowering. Look at how he's grieving.

Now imagine that the Hassan who believes that your younger brother is alive also steps out of you and stands opposite you, next to the first Hassan. Look at him standing there, unencumbered and full of hope, in calm anticipation of seeing his brother again one day. Look at him, with all his power and vitality!

Now imagine that another Hassan steps out of him to the side – the Hassan who looks at the matter from every angle, who doubts, weighs things up and debates with himself: is it this way or that way? What is the truth, and how can I find assurance that it is the truth?

These three Hassans are standing over there. Look at them and how completely different they are. I'm going to ask you to talk to them from time to time, sometimes with the first Hassan, sometimes with the second, and sometimes with the third. Each of them is entitled to your attention, but since they're so different, you should talk to each of the three Hassans in the way that is right for him. I'm sure you get what I'm driving at – not at the same time, but in rotation."

Hassan looked relieved and said that he liked that idea. The course of therapy continued for a while longer, but he no longer raised the matter of his brother.[62]

Dividing up the ex-husband

It is not only ourselves that we can divide up into several different persons, but also our internal image of other individuals. I suggested the following to a woman who had been left by her husband Dieter (not his real name) for another woman, and who lamented that she was still in love with him, even though there was no hope that he would ever return to her.

"Imagine taking your internal image of Dieter out of your head and putting him over there for now. Is that OK?

Now imagine dividing him up into several different people. On the left we'll put the Dieter who is bad for you, who betrayed you, whom you'd like to give a good kicking, and whose departure is no great loss. Can you imagine him?

To the right of him now is the remainder of Dieter, who's actually OK, and perhaps even better than OK. Can you see him there as well?

Now let's divide that Dieter in two again. Second from the left we'll put the one who I'm going to say is like a bottle of red wine – dreaming of him is as pleasurable as knocking back glass after glass, but then the next morning comes and you wake up and think, 'Oh no, he left me!' And then you feel awful. The Dieter who only makes you feel good if you are dreaming of him, and then bad when you wake up from the dream, is no good for you overall. He can go second from the left. Is that OK?

And now on the far right is the Dieter who stands for everything that is good for you in the long term, and whom you can think about without it hurting. You can take this Dieter with you.

Now we can open the door. To the Dieter on the far left, you can say, 'Time's up. I don't need you any more. Go in peace, but go!'

To the one second from the left, you can say, 'You're another one who's no good for me. And I don't need you any more either. Go, but go in peace!' To the one on the right, you can say, 'You can stay!' How does that seem to you?"[63]

The woman was amenable to the suggestion, seemed relieved and moved onto other topics during the rest of the conversation.

Dividing something up into multiple "people" also works even if the stress is not embodied by a real person.

Separating symptoms and values

"Imagine that the person who has osteoarthrosis in her shoulder and is therefore familiar with this pain and limited mobility could step out of you and go and stand over there. How do you think she'd look?

Let's imagine dividing her in two; we'll put the one with symptoms on the left, and the one who has good intentions and probably simply hasn't found a better way to achieve them than with osteoarthritis, on the right. Now that's someone with real values! How does she look? What do you think might be her good intentions and her values?

I think that values are always good. Is it OK with you if the one on the right returns to you and steps back inside you again?

What exactly has happened in terms of the pain you were previously feeling? And how about the mobility of your arm?"

Clients who put this intervention to the test in therapy typically report that the pain has significantly diminished or disappeared entirely, and that they can move their arm more easily. The change is generally long-lasting. In order to ensure that this is the case, however, it is a good idea to stabilise the outcome yet further. The influence of objections raised by internal and external sceptics is lessened since the therapist presents the effectiveness of the intervention as plausible and makes the concerns seem implausible, or honours their good intention and makes a distinction between this good intention and their inopportune suggestive effects.

In the context of grief, we can therefore also dissociate from the client and from each other "the person who has symptoms of grief" and "the grieving person who has values". The client can test out how it feels to be linked to the values (love, loyalty) and how it feels to differentiate herself from the symptoms of grief (pain, insomnia). This new condition can then be further stabilised, for example using the methods of therapeutic modelling and therapeutic greetings.

If my memory serves me well, the grieving people with whom I have tried out this approach have without exception experienced it as a huge relief.

If from the outset we see the persons subject to a burden who have been dissociated from an individual not as "parts of a personality", but instead as opportunities for experiences or as options that the unconscious can realise or otherwise, then it is also possible to bid farewell to these persons, with all due esteem (and with remarkable impacts on clients' experiences).

Letting genies out of bottles

"Let's imagine for now that the invisible people here are genies in bottles, of the sort you find in the Arabian Nights. If we let a genie of this kind out of its bottle, it will typically say something along the lines of, 'Thank you for releasing me. I've been trapped in this bottle for one hundred years. Now I can return home to the kingdom from which I come. If you ever need me, simply call on me and I will be of service to you!' You can say to the genie, 'I'll call on you if I need you, and if I don't call on you I won't need you. Go in peace!' Then the genie disappears into thin air. Imagine that the people we've imagined now gradually fade further and further away until they've disappeared. Now you and I are alone in the room. How does that feel?"

Almost all clients find this idea extremely liberating and beneficial. And if someone feels the opposite, all we need to do is to summon the genie back again, and it will return in the blink of an eye!

2.3.3 Bringing solution-oriented persons into play

Instead of projecting imagined persons who are subject to a particular burden out of a client and onto a place in the room, it is possible for the helpful persons they could potentially be to be placed in the room and summoned into the client following a description of their physiological appearance. In keeping with the principle of "linking solutions", we do this with figures who are associated with resources, skills, or solutions, or in other words the client's target experience.

A client who observes an individual of this kind will build up a rapport with this internal image. Her facial expressions, gestures, breathing, movements etc. will increasingly resemble those of this figure, while she …

- describes this person,
- becomes curious about whether she will in fact feel like this person when she's there,
- sits in her place and notices for herself what is different there,
- makes a distinction between the person in the previous place and herself in the new place.

These changes can also be identified directly from the client's altered physiology during the process.

It is furthermore possible to transform figures who are subject to a burden[64] into figures whose burden has been relieved. It is also worth considering "the client who you were when you came here, who is sitting in the previous place before our inner eye" for this purpose. One option for transforming problem-associated figures into solution-associated figures is the heavenly journey.[65] The use of clones is another possibility.

A liberating clone

"Imagine that while you're sitting here and noticing how much better you feel, we could ask your clone to step out of you – a second person identical to you – and she could divide herself up into several more clones identical to you, and we could ask her to feel just as good and even better while she goes and stand over there, exactly where the stressed-out people who stepped out of you beforehand are standing, and to update their systems so that they feel as good as you do. In my imagination I see something like a green progress bar that gets longer and longer, 1%, 2%, 3%, etc., all the way up to 100%. Now look at how these people are sitting there differently, and how different they look! Can you describe it to me? A clone can also go over to the one you were when you were sitting on that chair before, and fill her up with your good experience. Look at her now. How has she changed?"

In order to transform persons suffering from stress or sceptical persons into helpful figures, they can be entrusted – once they have been dissociated from the client – with a new task by means of which they can support her more effectively. A person who raises objections to the effectiveness of therapy can be acknowledged for having wanted to avoid disappointment, but at the same time alerted to the fact that she is likely to be achieving precisely what she wanted to avoid through the mechanism of a self-fulfilling prophecy. She can be offered a job as a scientific observer or as a Minister for Confidence[66] in the client's life.[67]

2.3.4 The transgenerational perspective

If we ask clients, "How long have you had this problem?", they sometimes answer, "always". This sounds like a vague response, but in fact it typically gets right to the heart of the matter. If we continue to ask, "Around the time of your birth – immediately at the time of your birth or in the six months before or after – was there anything special going on in your family?", then we often hear about circumstances with a high potential for trauma. In many cases the client's voice, fluency of speaking, and visible physiology also express stress while they are discussing the subject.

Some clients explain that they were born prematurely and spent the first few weeks of their lives in an incubator, whereas others say that they were unwanted or perhaps even that their mothers had considered aborting them. Others talk about how they were given away by their parents, how their mother was depressed or how their parents were barely able to care for a baby because they were struggling with a bereavement or working all hours.

This might perhaps be an adequate explanation for why long-term physical and mental problems have emerged. Yet if we are not satisfied with this explanation and continue to ask, "Did either of your parents have similar symptoms?", astonishingly often the answer is in the affirmative. If we then continue to ask, "Do you have any idea what the origin of that might have been for your mother (or your father)?", reference is sometimes made to a stressful experience, often in their childhood. It often transpires that a parent of this parent was already very familiar with the same behaviour and experience described as problematic. Sometimes the phenomenon can also be traced back another few generations. It is also not uncommon for queries about the origins of the problem to lead back to ancestors about whom precise details are no longer passed on within the family (at least not verbally). Based on my observations, in the case of women such transfers most often follow the line "mother/grandmother/great-grandmother", whereas in the case of men they frequently follow the line "father/grandfather/great-grandfather", although it is of course possible for them to trace out a genealogical zigzag.

For many years, debate raged among those seeking to understand how patterns of problems (e.g. depressive behaviour and experiences) are passed on from generation to generation, with the debate centring on the question of what is responsible for this phenomenon – "genetic" factors or "acquired" factors. Vulnerability concepts were developed, according to which a genetic predisposition to certain stresses exists in some families that is "expanded" by certain biographical experiences, meaning that the body takes the step from the potential for a symptom to a symptom that is specifically experienced. In systemic therapy and in work with system constellations, familial patterns are often interpreted as being stored in the collective conscious or unconscious of a family or group. This approach is explained sometimes in neurobiological terms (the phenomenon of mirror neurons, which allow individuals in a group to create a shared experience involuntarily), sometimes in spiritual terms (drawing on an invisible well of knowledge), and sometimes also in terms of quantum physics phenomena (the physical storage of information in a manner not dependent on space or time).[68]

The field of epigenetics research gives rise to new interpretative possibilities for the transgenerational transfer of information within a family (and sometimes beyond the boundaries of an individual family).

For example, a mental trauma does not only trigger an immediate and severe stress and fear reaction in the body. If it occurs repeatedly or is particularly intense, it also changes the epigenomes (*molecular structures attached to strands of DNA that turn genes on and off*) in the cells of the brain and the hormone system that trigger fear or determine the sensitivity of stress regulation. As a result, the way in which our body and mind respond to comparable situations in the future also changes. An epigenetic adaptation of this kind can then sometimes be observable even decades later. If it is furthermore passed on to subsequent generations via the germ line, it changes even the biology of these descendants (at least theoretically). We are thus epigenetically shaped over the course of our own life and by the lifestyle and experiences of our ancestors. Our personality and susceptibility to disease are therefore not just a question of the genes we have inherited, but without exception also a question of the way in which the past has shaped us epigenetically.[69]

Experiments investigating transgenerational epigenetics have been carried out using rats and mice in particular, but also other vertebrates, insects, worms, and plants. The specific epigenetic alterations observed in the sperm of traumatised mice and rats were also seen in the same form or a modified form in their children and grandchildren. The rodents with trauma-specific alterations to their epigenome similar to those observed in their parents exhibited depressed behaviour and pronounced social anxieties, even if neither they nor their mother had ever met the traumatised father (IVF conception). "Some of the symptoms exhibited by the dysfunctional mice also have a very prominent presence in patients diagnosed with borderline personality disorder, depression or schizophrenia."[70] It was possible for the effects described to be traced down the generations to grandchildren or sometimes even great-grandchildren.[71] The epigenetic "inheritance of the consequences of trauma [demonstrably] follows either the paternal or the maternal line; in both cases, the germ cells are involved."[72]

In the case of animals which had suffered trauma and which were then placed in a very positively stimulating environment with playmates, toys, and lots of opportunities for movement (as "therapy"), the behaviours typical of depression and social phobia gradually disappeared, as did the corresponding epigenetic structures. Their descendants also behaved like members of the same species who had grown up normally and had an epigenome typical of the species. The special epigenetic features remained stable in animals raised in a more neutral environment after suffering a trauma, and they passed them on to their descendants.[73]

In other experimental configurations, the rodents that had "inherited" traumatic information from their father or their mother in this way were particularly resistant to stress or particularly goal-oriented and flexible.[74] In one experiment (which has not yet been validated by subsequent experiments), mice were taught to fear the smell of cherry blossom, and this fear was passed on to the next generation.[75]

In order to explore whether these results are applicable to humans, two researchers – Elisabeth Binder and Rachel Yehuda – investigated the genetic material of 32 Jewish Holocaust survivors and compared it to the DNA of Jews of the same age who had not endured the Holocaust. The capacity for activation of a specific gene for stress regulation was altered much more frequently in the Holocaust victims than in the comparison group. This means that the relevant individual's sensitivity to stress is reduced (in both humans and animals). The epigenomes of the children of these Holocaust survivors exhibited a clearly increased capacity for activation of the stress regulation gene at the same point, meaning that they tended to be prone to stress. According to Binder, this is,

> a potential explanation for why the risk of stress-related diseases such as depression, bipolar diseases or anxiety disorders is raised in the ancestors of Holocaust survivors. [...] We were specifically able to rule out other influences, for example new traumas in early childhood.[76]

Comparable outcomes were achieved by studies involving women who had survived the genocide in Rwanda and their children. Both the epigenome of the relevant women and the epigenome of their descendants exhibited trauma-specific changes.[77] The outcome of an epigenetic study of blood cells from adolescents aged between 10 and 19 whose mothers had been abused by their partners during pregnancy was basically the same.[78]

Spork summarises the situation as follows; "The fact that we humans can therefore pass on our traumas to our descendants has therefore been established for the most part. The question as to the precise mechanisms that are responsible for this remains open, however." Potential causes include both, "transfer via the germ line, as in mice and other laboratory animals, and also increased levels of stress hormones or the behaviour of parents during the child's perinatal development phase."[79]

Conversely, it is also true that epigenetic structures that are apparently trauma-based and that result in mentally stressful experiences can be scaled back. For example, researchers studying the blood cells of 28 patients suffering from frequent panic attacks discovered a certain epigenetic alteration in a specific gene that is often activated particularly strongly in patients with experience of panic attacks.

Following six weeks of cognitive behavioural therapy, some of the patients had stopped suffering from panic attacks, and the relevant epigenetic signature had also disappeared in these patients … The epigenetic markers had become even more distinctive in patients whose therapy had failed, however.[80]

Notes

1 For further details of the intertwining of physical and psychological experiences, see Hammel 2019a, 15 *et seqq.*, Hammel 2011, 50 *et seqq.*
2 Schmidt 2009.
3 Hammel 2020, 67 et seqq. Unterberger, Wilcke and Witt (2014) note the following: "A number of different studies testify to the fact that individuals with an increased potential for anxiety also tend to suffer from allergic reactions." See Balon 2006. A recent analysis of 4,181 test subjects revealed that densensitisation treatment had at least influenced the state of mind of persons suffering from allergies to the extent that their psychiatric anxiety and depression diagnoses had declined significantly. See Goodwin et al. 2012, Roy-Byrne et al. 2008. If the time-consuming course of treatment produces its effect via psychological factors, a psychological intervention would certainly be a more direct, simple, effective and cheap means." Unterberger et al. 2014, 23. The authors refer to case studies in which allergic reactions occurred for the first time directly in traumatic situations or situations involving conflict and persisted until a course of therapy involving consideration of psychological factors. See ibid., 23 *et seqq.* The doctor Salomon Sellam describes a large number of medical case studies that point to the fact that traumatic experiences ("psy-choc émotionel déstabilisant") might trigger long-term allergic reactions: "Dans la quasi-totalité des histoires d'allergie il existe un … episode [destabilisant à l'origine du déclenchement des symptomes] plus ou moins occulté aujourd'hui." According to Sellam, the allergen is directly associated with a dangerous situation which is being ignored and for which it serves as a warning: "L'allergéne … est toujours accolé à une situation de danger précédemment ressenti comme telle … L'allergéne n'est qu'un simple avertisseur de l'imminence d'un danger dèjà connu, mais occulté." See Sellam 2006, 37 *et seqq.*
Gunther Schmidt refers to the "somatopsychological" nature of allergies. See Schmidt 2009.
4 The deconstruction of phobic structures by means of "flooding" is not recommended because the method involves a comparatively large amount of suffering compared to other effective options and is potentially retraumatising.
5 It is not only visual errors or auditory "filling in the gaps" when listening to an MP3 (a lossy data-compressed file) that can be categorised in this manner, but also immunological mistakes in connection with autoimmune diseases.
6 Watzlawick et al. 2011, 130 et passim.
7 Schmidt 2004, 233, 238 *et seqq.*, *passim.*

8 Zeig 1982, vii. In Greek mythology, Procrustes would welcome overnight guests with open arms. Once evening came, he would lead them to an iron bed made to the dimensions of his own body. If the guests were too big for the bed, he would amputate their limbs; if they were too small, he would stretch them lengthwise. All that mattered was that they should fit in his bed.

9 Schmidt 2004, 183.

10 See the case study in Hammel 2019a, 56 *et seq.*

11 Hammel 2019a, 52 *et seqq.*

12 Schmidt 2004, 183 *et seqq.*; see Meiss 2016, 87 *et seqq.*; Muffler 2015, 15. For illustrative examples of problem trances and their "dehypnosis" or transformation into solution trances, see Bierbaum-Luttermann & Mrochen 2019, 14 *et seqq.*, *passim.*

13 "One cannot not communicate" is one of Paul Watzlawick's key axioms. Watzlawick goes further by criticising the viewpoint that "manipulation" is firstly bad, and secondly avoidable: "It is difficult to imagine how *any* behavior in the presence of another person can avoid being a communication of one's own view of the nature of one's relationship with that person and how it can, therefore, fail to influence that person ... the problem therefore, is not how influence and manipulation can be avoided, but how they can best be comprehended and used in the interest of the patient." Watzlawick et al. 2011, xix. See Muffler 2015, 15: "Suggestions are an everyday and unavoidable component of communication – not only the communication that takes place between different individuals, but also the communication that takes place as an individual's internal dialogue."

14 Schmidt 2005, 67.

15 See Schmidt 2004, 69: "While speaking to me, Erickson emphasised that in over 50 years of professional practice he had always worked consistently in a hypnotherapeutic style, but that no more than 25% of his work had used direct trance inductions that were 'officially' defined as such. [These inductions] ... are therefore only a special case of flexible, context-dependent hypnotherapy."

16 See the concept of infectious health, Hammel 2012c, 51; Hammel 2019a, 38 *et seq.* For further details of the construction of plausibility, see section "Factors affecting therapy", Factors 2 and 3 in this chapter,

17 For further details of the generation of reality through the focusing of attention, see Domanski 2022, 34 *et seqq.*

18 For details of the focusing of attention through dissociation and association, see "Separating, linking and transforming" in this chapter and section (Assumptions and attitudes from hypnotherapy).

19 "In this way ... internal and external images, kinaesthetic, gustatory and olfactory impressions, experiences of age and size, breathing patterns and bodily coordination are linked with behaviour, judgements and the attribution of meaning. Linkages of this kind are referred to as 'patterns'. Experience is the outcome of patterns of this kind that are assembled by the individual (on a voluntary and involuntary level)." See Schmidt 2005, 181.

20 For further details of pacing ambivalences, see Schmidt 2005, 85 *et seqq.*

21 For further details of utilisation, see the section on systemic therapy, "Utilisation (use everything!)" in this chapter. See also Hammel 2011; Hammel 2012b; Hammel 2016c and Short & Weinspach 2007, 239 *et seqq.*

22 Erickson 1959, 3 *et seq.*, 20.

23 The possibilities of multi-level communication are explored in detail in Hammel 2014a.

24 Peyton 2017, 31 with a reference to Lieberman et al. 2011 and Coan et al. 2006. Lieberman and his team were able to demonstrate the effectiveness of this procedure using imaging techniques (brain fMRI).

25 "Since – as we know – all experience is the result of focusing attention, the speed and effectiveness with which the desired goals can be achieved depends on the extent to

which the details of the relevant experience are described in a differentiated manner. That allows the individual to focus on them and imagine them, which in turn is what makes them realisable in the first place." Schmidt 2005, 102.

26 Actions are symbolic in the narrower sense if they achieve something figuratively (e.g. lighting a candle to commemorate something), and metonymic if they achieve a part that is representative of the whole ("*pars pro toto*", e.g. laying a foundation stone).

27 One intervention that pursues this goal is "The earth rotates forwards" in Chapter 8, section "Therapeutic greetings" and another is the anecdote "On the side turned towards me" in Chapter 9, section "Dispelling doubts and creating optimism".

28 See section "Abandonment and Trauma" in Chapter 3.

29 Ibid. ("Triggers").

30 See the exercise "Taking one's own history" at the start of Chapter 7.

31 "When emotional experience has not yet been named it is still present in the body … And it is possible to still feel anxious and ashamed when thinking of childhood pain, even after seventy years have passed. When the emotion is finally known and named, it is possible for the body-brain can begin to relax into the message received by the brain in the skull. Peyton 2017, 37. Both are important – jointly examining and acknowledging burdensome experiences *and* regulating the emotional pain that arises in the work, through empathetic support, reframing, a new dissociation, simultaneous examination and distraction or working "one-step removed" by addressing the problem indirectly. See Hammel 2011, 144; Zeig 1985, 50, 64.

32 See Alexander Hartmann, Die Hypnose Revolution, www.alexander hartmann.de/kostenlos.

33 Domanski 2022, 39, emphases by the author.

34 See the observation made by Gunther Schmidt: "Body coordination apparently serves as a strong attractor in the experience pattern, in that it 'attracts' the other involuntary pattern elements. There are no exceptions to the rule that, 'What you put in is what you get out …' Although you might initially have to 'fake it until you make it,' assuming the body coordination experienced as conducive to the goal at the same time as experiencing a symptom will typically result in an extremely beneficial shift after a relatively short period of time." Schmidt 2005, 115.

35 Hammel 2019b, 26 *et seq.*; Domanski 2022, 48 *et seqq.*

36 See Schweitzer & Schlippe 2007, 83; Hammel 2019a, 144 *et seq.*

37 Schmidt 2004, 65; see Schmidt in Leeb et al. 2011, 18 *et seqq.*

38 The sentence can be useful in many different life situations; it was said by a patient diagnosed with psychosis when he noticed how his delusion of entering hell had eased. See Hammel 2016b, 61.

39 Schmidt 2005, 86.

40 For further details of utilisation as the central approach and methodology of systems therapy and hypnotherapy and the development of problem and solution models for individual therapy, see Hammel 2011 and Hammel 2012b. Details of the technique of reframing can be found in the section on systemic therapy, "Utilisation" in this chapter. See also Hammel 2011, 245 *et seqq.*; Hammel 2019a, 226 *et seqq.*

41 The intervention dissuaded a Polish nature lover who was living in Germany from his plan of committing suicide.

42 See also the intervention "The four quadrants" in section "Therapeutic spaces" under the heading "Spatial area models".

43 See also the intervention "Ordeal" in Chapter 9, section on "Dispelling doubts and building optimism".

44 Claudia Weinspach in Hammel et al. 2020, 13 *et seq.*; see Bierbaum-Luttermann & Mrochen 2019, 18: "Social phobias lead to a permanently restricted awareness of self, for example through the focus on 'others' views of oneself that are assumed to be

negative'. Anorexic and also depressed adolescents turn their knowledge, their intelligence and ultimately also their interests against themselves and use their fantasy and imagination – largely unconsciously – to manoeuvre ever deeper into the quagmire of their negative mental states. This means that experiences of this kind are reproduced again and again."

45 Saint-Exupéry 2017, 41.
46 See Hammel 2012c, 57.
47 For further details of the concept of therapeutic double binds, see Erickson et al.1976, 62 et seqq., 69f., 63f.; Hammel 2011, 218 *et seqq.*; Short & Weinspach 2007, 246 *et seqq.*
48 See the section on systemic therapy, "Asking good questions" in this chapter and Chapter 7, section on systemic questions.
49 For further details of reframing, see Schlippe & Schweitzer 1996, 177 *et seqq.*; Mücke 1998, 314 *et seqq.*; Hammel 2019a, 226 *et seqq.* and Hammel 2011, 247 *et seqq.* A collection of reframings that are suitable for universal application is provided by Prior 2017.
50 Hammel 2012c, 63.
51 Hammel 2019a, 236 *et seqq.*; Hammel 2011, 210 *et seq.*, 247 *et seqq.*, 270 *passim*; Mücke 1998, 319 *et seqq.*, 410.
52 Schmidt 2004, 58 *et seqq.*, 93 *passim.*
53 See Chapter 8, section "Therapeutic stories" and section "Therapeutic maps and landscapes".
54 The following address systemic question formats in detail: Schlippe & Schweitzer 1996, 137 *et seqq.*, 263 *et seqq.*; Mücke 1998, 279 *et seqq.*; Simon & Rech-Simon 2000.
55 See Schmidt 2005, 82 *et seq.*: "Questions are of pivotal importance in terms of how the system might organise itself so that it can operate in an optimally productive manner: 'How would the system need to organise itself – around the goals, so to speak – so that it furthers these goals particularly effectively and rapidly?'"
56 In-depth reflections on the implications of questions can be found in Hammel 2014a, 255 et seqq.
57 The miracle question emerged in the 1980s as part of the solution-focused brief therapy developed by Steve de Shazer and Insoo Kim Berg, see Shazer & Dolan 2021, 70.
58 See the section on hypnotherapy, "Factors affecting therapy" in this chapter, Factor 5.
59 Ibid, Factor 4.
60 See Chapter 8, section "Therapeutic greetings".
61 See the section on psychodrama, constellation work and parts work in this chapter as well as Chapter 7, section on life opportunities and Chapter 8, section "Therapeutic modelling". A detailed description of therapeutic modelling can be found in Hammel 2019b.
62 A further intervention that was used in relation to this issue with the same client can be found in Hammel et al. 2021, p. 60 *et seq.*
63 The intervention is also described in Hammel et al. 2021, p. 61 *et seq.*
64 Remember the "I" who is "many"…
65 Outlined in the section on psychodrama, constellation work and parts work, "Inside and outside" in this chapter.
66 Hammel 2020, 31 *et seq.*
67 See Chapter 9, section "Dispelling doubts and building optimism".
68 For further details of the identification of transgenerational stresses and the relevant therapy, see the section on psychodrama, parts, and constellation work, "The transgenerational perspective" in this chapter as well as Chapter 7, section on the use of life opportunities, "Transgenerational history-taking".
69 Spork 2017, 357.

70 The Zurich-based neuroepigeneticist Isabelle Mansuy, quoted in Spork 2017, 270. 89
    Ibid., 149 *et seq.*, 269 *et seqq.*
71 Ibid., 149 *et seq.*, 269 *et seqq.*
72 Mansuy et al. 2020, 131.
73 Spork 2017, 274, Mansuy et al. 2020, 137; Gapp et al. 2016.
74 Spork 2017, 143 *et seq.*, 273 *et seq.*; Mansuy et al. 2020, 134 *et seq.*
75 Spork 2017, 275.
76 Ibid., 282 *et seqq.*; see R. Yehuda et al. 2016.
77 Mansuy et al. 2020, 92.
78 Spork 199 *et seq.*
79 Ibid., 284 *et seq.*
80 Ibid., 57 *et seq.* with a reference to Ziegler et al. 2016.

Part 2

What hurts us and what heals us

It is in relationships that we are wounded, but it is only in relationships that we become whole again.

There is a passage in the Bible that talks about how people try to shape their relationships without acting in accordance with the values they experience. In my opinion, it holds true regardless of your religion or ideology:

> If I speak in the tongues of men or of angels, but do not have love, I am only a resounding gong or a clanging cymbal.
>
> If I have the gift of prophecy and can fathom all mysteries and all knowledge, and if I have a faith that can move mountains, but do not have love, I am nothing.
>
> If I give all I possess to the poor and give over my body to hardship that I may boast, but do not have love, I gain nothing.[1]

We could adapt this to a modern context by saying,

> If I complete training in all the schools of therapy and learn an infinite number of techniques, so that my counselling toolbox is overflowing, but I do not live a life based on compassion, acceptance, respect, and recognition, I gain nothing.

Assuming a respectful, caring, and considerate attitude, and searching for the legitimate needs and good intentions behind everything – consciously and subconsciously, secretly and in public, where people will hear it and where no one can see it – is more important than all the models and techniques in the world if we wish to help individuals experience themselves as healed. And yet it is also true that whoever adopts an attitude of facilitating clients almost unconditionally[2] *while at the same time* searching for, finding and refining helpful models and techniques will achieve yet more again than someone who dedicates his life to love without tools of this kind.

The following chapter outlines models that have proven helpful as a guide to therapeutic approaches in a world of suffering that is associated on a mental, physical, social, and sometimes also intercultural and global level.

DOI: 10.4324/9781003425014-4

Notes

1 1. Cor. 13, 1–3, New International Version.
2 For Erickson, utilisation means "an initial acceptance of the patient's presenting behavior by the operator, however seemingly adverse that presenting behavior may appear to be in the clinical situation." Erickson 1959, 3 *et seq.*

Chapter 3

Looking backwards and looking forwards

In any living system a balance is struck between different tendencies, namely those that are aimed at ...

*   stabilising it, or in other words the maintenance of a status quo,
*   expanding it, or in other words growth and reproduction, or
*   changing it, or in other words adapting to a shifting environment.

In order for a living system to be able to provide for itself and reproduce, it therefore creates for itself self-reflexive rules that are the only thing allowing it to rebuild itself and that are also intended – among other things – to ensure that the rules themselves continue to be kept in place. Since this in turn happens in confrontation with an environment in a constantly fluctuating state of change, however, it is not enough to leave all of the previous rules rigidly in place (homeostasis); instead, the system must also repeatedly change some of the rules to reflect the environment, with the specific aim of ensuring that its stability continues to be possible; "Anyone who wants to remain more or less the same must constantly change."[1]

3.1 Role and identity

What, if anything, is "identical" about our identity? Identity is the flip side of role, or in other words our place within the system (our herd and our or their territory). We experience identity when our view of ourselves and other key individuals' view of us coincide for the most part.[2] Alongside this interpersonal definition, an intrapersonal definition is also possible: we experience identity when our self-description represents a continuum, or in other words when we experience our view of ourselves in the recent past and in the here and now as consistent. This implies that what we call identity is not innate for the most part, and neither does it remain the same for a lifetime; instead, it is subject to change. All that exists is our body's psychobiological functions, which promote a stable experience of self through the paradigmatic repetition of behaviours and interpretations, through the relativisation

DOI: 10.4324/9781003425014-5

(e.g. forgetting) of differences between earlier and current experience and through the reinterpretation of change in oneself as change in the environment.

> Depending on where focus is currently directed (or in other words on which of the many possible areas of experience), we become someone else in part, since one of the many possible versions of our personality effectively leaps into our consciousness and takes on the "governing role"... We are so to speak non-existent as static beings; in reality, our experience involves being rein-vented and regenerated second by second through the focusing of our attention. Hypnotherapy merely takes advantage of these processes ... This is not a new discovery, however. All shamanic healing procedures ... adhere to the same principle ...: "Energy flows where attention goes ..." Similarly, physiology, emotion and thinking are realised where attention goes.[3]

Based on Reinhold Bartl's work, Cordula Meyer-Erben and Ute Zander-Schreindorfer differentiate between two options for focusing attention.

> a desired direction, in which well-being, satisfaction, coherence or a feeling of flow arise, or an undesired direction, which is perceived as a problem or which is exhibited in the symptom behaviour with an experience of suffering. Both levels each have a special wealth of knowledge that we can use in the search for solutions.[4]

In this connection, Bartl refers to three authorities or sources of knowledge that focus our attention:

> the conscious "I", the involuntary "it" and the body. The conscious "I" can be described as our conscious thinking; it encompasses our image of ourselves with all our strengths, weaknesses, conscious values etc. – and the "I want (for good reasons) world" of rationality. The involuntary "It" encompasses feelings and impulses that arise involuntarily – the "it happens/feels (for good reasons) world" of intuition. The third authority is the body, which was referred to by the leading brain researcher Antonio Damasio as the stage of feelings. The body responds to the impulses of the involuntary "it".[5]

3.1.1 A place in the herd

The British anthropologist and psychologist Robin Dunbar explains the evolution of language in the early days of the human race as communicative "grooming" in large social structures. In his opinion, gossip has been the cement holding groups together since the dawn of mankind. In that respect, according to the historian Yuval Harari,

> our language evolved as a way of gossiping ... *Homo sapiens* is primarily a social animal. Social cooperation is our key for survival and reproduction. It

is not enough for individual men and women to know the whereabouts of lions and bison. It's much more important for them to know who in their band hates whom, who is sleeping with whom, who is honest, and who is a cheat ... Reliable information about who could be trusted meant that small bands could expand into larger bands, and Sapiens could expand tighter and more sophisticated types of cooperation.[6]

If everyone in a group has roughly the same opinion about the others and if as many people as possible have roughly the same opinion of themselves as the others, it is easier to resolve questions of rank amicably than if insurmountable differences exist between group members in terms of their interpretation of the hierarchical situation. This reduces the potential for conflicts of rivalry. It is therefore likely that what we refer to as gossip furthers the goal of collectively adapting a group's images of itself and others, i.e. approximating intersubjectively ascribed roles and subjectively experienced identities within a group structure.

When a child comes into the world, he gets to know his mother, father, siblings, grandparents, and other attachment figures, and involuntarily develops models of their behaviour and their meaning within his life. His image of who he is himself can only be developed in the mirror of his treatment by others. What others say to him and how they treat him is essentially his only source of information about the place assigned to him within the system. His identity therefore becomes everything assigned to him by the key individuals in his environment, provided that he does not raise any objections.

What options does a child have to object to the way in which he is viewed and described and shaped by others? It is likely to be true that the place taken up by a child within a family is largely assigned to him by those who have already been part of the system for a long time. The severity or otherwise of the rules imposed on the younger generation by the elder members of a family or society as a whole is regulated differently in different families and different societies. The place in the herd is repeatedly renegotiated or fought over; this is typically a frequent phenomenon between siblings, but tends to take place in phases or waves between children and grown-ups.

> Individual experiential and behavioural processes are therefore also interpreted as phenomena which take place in networks of interactions, and which are affected by the way in which these rules are regulated. They can no longer merely be described on the basis of observations by the "I", the "self", etc. ... Every behaviour by every participant is simultaneously the cause and effect of the behaviour of the other participants (circularity). It thus also makes little sense to define particular "character traits", for example to say that a person "is" such and such; instead, their "being such and such" is comprehended as part of a process of interdependency and as part of an interaction in their systemic context.[7]

A person can experience great confusion if his entire system behaves as though certain things were facts when these facts are contradicted by the actual situation, in a manner that is not down to individual interpretation. The person in question experiences a conflict between the construction of reality believed or prescribed by the surrounding system and the information provided by his own body, associated with a vague feeling of incongruence: "Something's not right here." A situation of this kind can arise if ...

- left-handed individuals are treated as though they were right-handed,
- girls are treated as though they were boys or the other way round,
- a child is treated as though he or she were someone else ("you're just like your dead brother/your grandmother"),
- expectant parents believed that *one* child was on the way, it turned out to be twins and the parents found it very difficult to adjust to the situation,
- a child was given no information or incorrect information about his biological parents (or one parent) and thus about all of his relatives,
- a child that is less gifted in certain areas is treated as extremely gifted, or the other way round,
- a child with homosexual leanings is told that there's no such thing as being gay or that being gay is reprehensible, etc.

Since we belong to different groups that assign different roles and different identifying features to us, we have different identities or states of being – including different behaviours and experiences – depending on the environment in which we operate.[8] This difference – experienced from an internal or external perspective – can be extremely discreet or very obvious. What can be described from the external perspective as a conflict of roles can typically also be described as a conflict between different identities.

If our experience of identity in different systems is difficult to reconcile or cannot be reconciled at all, we experience ourselves as being in conflict whenever these systems collide. This is particularly true if the systems impose demands on us at the same time, meaning that we must opt for one of the identities assigned to us and accepted by us, at the cost of the other identity.

When a child comes into the world, he is wholly dependent on those who care for him. Having a place in the herd is essential for survival. If we are not someone about whom things are told and to whom characteristics, skills, relationships, and special features are attributed, we experience ourselves as insignificant. *Belonging to a herd on the basis of give-and-take relationships is the biological essence of experiencing meaning. If we do not belong, we cannot experience meaning.*

The experience of belonging *is* the experience of meaning, or in other words: people are willing to make huge adjustments to their behaviour – even if these adjustments are sometimes horrifying, cause harm to others or themselves or seem ridiculous, and even if they involve correcting perception and memories – in order to experience a sense of belonging to others, in particular those who provide them with safety and a high status. This has been clearly demonstrated by the experiments carried out by Solomon Asch and Stanley Milgram[9] as well as the Stanford prison experiment by Philip Zimbardo.[10] This is also what happens when a distinction is drawn between the individual or group and others who allegedly have a lower status (aggressive nationalism, racism, homophobia, devaluation of the other sex etc.). In human societies, the distinction between "good" and "bad" ("evil", "inferior") is almost exclusively based on the relevant definition of the boundaries of "us" (people with the shared status features) and "them" (people with recognisably different status features). The opposite also applies: anyone who asks for the life story of people with the symptoms of depression will typically hear about emotional neglect, feeling unwelcome, or disrupted relationships in early childhood.

How is it that some people insult and disparage themselves? That can't be a good thing, after all – and yet it must perform a function.

In case of doubt, people assume any assigned identity if no other seems to be available, or in other words any position in the system that is associated with certain ways of behaving and experiencing. The general impression one receives is that, "any identity is better than none at all".

Supposing that a father hits his child and swears at him, and the child defends himself by hitting and swearing back – there is a high likelihood that the child will be hit and sworn at even more violently. The child learns that things get even worse if he defends himself. He no longer defends himself, and instead complies. If he insists (quietly or loudly) that he is not the person as whom he is being treated, he will at the same time experience an incongruence between his father's view of him and his own view – an incongruence that makes it very difficult to experience consistency and guaranteed belonging.

In order to be able to experience belonging and identity in a system of this kind, the child must not only refrain from any external protests, but also internally agree to the role within the family demanded by the beatings and insults.

He thus develops not only an internal image of his father who beats, insults, and shames him, but also an own internal voice or figure with which he treats himself just as he was treated. The good intention of this person is to facilitate an experience of belonging and identity based on consistency with the role allocated by the father.

Yet our understanding of who we are is based not only on who we are in the system of others, but also on who we are in the system of the remaining inhabited and uninhabited world. We locate ourselves not only in relation to a herd within which we seek first belonging and then a good position, but also in relation to a territory within which we seek safety and good opportunities for development.

A failure to experience continuity in this respect also has a devastating impact on the experience of a stable identity that is perceived as coherent. The question "Who am I?" arises not only for those who do not have a consistent place within a group to which they feel they belong, but also for those who have been removed from their accustomed environment. We thus observe depression not only in those who, because of painful previous experiences, react with alarm to (or are "triggered" by) experiences of loss, loneliness, and exclusion, but also in many of those with experiences of migration.

This is all the more true if the emigration was experienced not as a voluntary decision by the individual, and if the option of returning to the home country has been ruled out. The complete overturning of a societal system within which people oriented themselves can have a highly disadvantageous impact in this connection. Examples of this include the collapse of the German Democratic Republic as a state and as a legal and societal system, the breakup of Yugoslavia and the division of Poland between the USSR and Hitler's Germany in the 20th century.

Border violations, changes in borders, and mergers of territories that have to be tolerated on a compulsory basis can also be a source of lasting irritation. The same applies to regional, family, or individual territories such as plots of land, apartments, offices, a seat in church or at the cinema claimed by an individual for himself, or the car that an individual drives.

People whose homes have been broken into can often be observed to respond in a traumatised manner, even if they were absent at the time of the break-in. Even individuals whose personal belongings have been stolen from their car or the luggage rack of their bike sometimes exhibit traumatic reactions.

Violations of a space experienced as a protected private sphere – within the family, with neighbours or at the workplace – can also be experienced as deeply distressing. In order to avoid border violations, territories are marked – with barriers, fences, doors, beach towels on sunbeds, cosmetic products around a new boyfriend's sink, etc.

The mime artist Samy Molcho has put forward the idea that tidying up is also a way of marking territory. The partner or the child of the person tidying up might then not mark anything using that method, but would instead typically choose to leave objects lying around as an alternative method. By leaving things lying around or tidying them up respectively, the partners are erasing the territorial markings left by the other, which is what leads to conflicts.[11]

Arguments about the right way of loading a dishwasher and discussions between drivers and passengers can probably also be explained in the same way.

This would take us back to the world of the herd and the world of roles and identities again. Can family members be "marked" in the same way as territory? Cats do that by rubbing their neck on people's legs and leaving behind a scent trail. Could a love bite perform a similar role? Buying clothing and jewellery for one's partner? A wedding ring? Can people be "marked" by uniforms and manners of dress?

Since we're talking about territorial marking, is there a "pecking order" in groups of humans? Can abuse that leaves behind bruises document one person's claim to ownership of another? The use of different types of violence or threats of violence in order to establish rank can often be observed in families and at workplaces. Salary bands and military ranks, as well as different models of company cars and differently decorated offices, can be regarded as attempts to make these rankings visible. At the same time, the official ranking does not always coincide with the informal and invisible order. Length of service, age, and – depending on culture – sex or a social status determined in a different way (aristocratic title, academic degree, caste) can also play a role in this connection.

Within a group that understands itself as an "us", rankings mark higher and lower gradings of people on a particular scale. Assigned identities also exist, e.g. "good" and "evil", "competent" and "incompetent", "healthy" and "sick", and often also "perpetrator" and "victim".

3.1.2 Perpetrators and victims

Therapists often tend to identify with individuals who perceive themselves as victims more than those who see themselves as perpetrators. Why is that the case? Are people who endure suffering better than those who inflict suffering? Is it important to identify the intention or need underlying the suffering inflicted by some and endured by others? Is it important to recognise whether and how they defend themselves? Is it relevant to know the back story and after story of the "perpetrators" and "victims" of violence?

When people have suffered, one must not take the side of the individual who has inflicted suffering on them. And yet sometimes it is possible, provided that we recognise the injustice that has been suffered, to say something to shift the architecture of interpretation in such a way that people are invited to move away from suffering and towards something more constructive …

What your mother did to you

"When I hear about what your parents did to you, I get quite cross. But if I had your mother here in therapy, she might tell me about what her mother did to her, and then I'd get cross at your grandmother. And if I had your grandmother here and she also told me about her mother, I'd get cross at your great-grandmother. So I think it might be better to say, 'I feel sad about what these people did and probably also suffered from doing.'"

My fear is that therapists who put themselves emphatically on the side of the individual who is suffering, and in the process take sides against the party who caused the suffering, may inadvertently invite their clients to remain on the side of those who are suffering or to move over imperceptibly to the side of those who inflict suffering on others, with the justification that they themselves have suffered. In training and supervisory settings, I therefore use a number of additional stories in order to invite therapists to examine the issue from many different angles.

Insects are creepy

I recall a conversation with a schoolgirl, who told me,

"I find insects creepy."
"Why?"

"They do really horrible things, like laying their eggs in other insects, so that mag-
  gots grow in them and eat them from the inside out. I can't even bear to
  think about it. But it doesn't bother my brother."
"And why doesn't it bother your brother?"
"He identifies with the insect that lays its eggs in other animals rather than with
  the animal that is eaten up."

The girl was not criticising her brother. She was merely pointing out a difference between them. I found that noteworthy.

Partisans

Partisans are hated by soldiers because they snipe at the enemy. That is seen as cowardly by the soldiers. Soldiers are hated by partisans because they come in large numbers. *That* is viewed as cowardly by the partisans. How someone fights depends on the opportunities available to them. Terrorists and freedom fighters are the same people. The difference between them depends on whose side you're on.

Cat and mouse

"God loves the cat and the mouse."[12]
   Time and again I find it necessary to move away from the "taking of sides" that results from empathy and to return to a position of multiple perspectives.
   Sometimes people talk about perpetrators and victims as though these epithets were facts or lasting identities, or something that could be unambiguously defined. Yet ...

A rose is a rose is a rose. A thistle is a thistle is a thistle. Blossoms and prickles. Who decides what is a plant, and what is a weed? Which criteria do they apply? If I mediate in a conflict – whose side am I on? That of the victims? What about if both sides believe that they are the victims?
   What about when the circle turns? The former victims are the current per- petrators who are the former victims. The former perpetrators are the current victims who are the former perpetrators. How many perpetrators are victims of perpetrators who are victims of perpetrators who are victims of perpetrators?
   How many victims remain victims or become perpetrators because being neither a victim nor a perpetrator and instead neither of the two would represent a loss of meaning in the shadow of suffering? How many victims atone end- lessly? Certain ways of supporting victims can mark the beginning of turning them into perpetrators. Who is to say that they will stop halfway and remain perpetrators of good? By fighting against perpetrators, I start to turn them into victims. Who is to say that *they* will stop halfway and stop doing evil if they suffer evil?
   What benefits one person harms another; what one person sees as praise, another sees as criticism; what helps one person is viewed as punishment by

another. It is only if the counsellor can break free from these thoughts that he can then break through the cycle of guilt. How can we succeed in doing so? Must the counsellor first come to terms with his own biography?[13]

Perpetrator, crime, and victim (The scissors)

Perhaps it is not about recognising that someone has been a victim, but that this individual has suffered and that this suffering came upon her undeservedly. Perhaps it is about decoupling her experience of identity and her life history from this suffering and from the life history of the "perpetrator". It would, however, be necessary to ensure that an additional burden was not placed on whomever had suffered beforehand, that what had happened was not trivialised and that demands were not placed on a client already suffering stress. Sometimes, when forgiveness is demanded, I feel like we are being asked to absolve the perpetrator of his responsibility.[14] If a thread attached the crime to the perpetrator, and another thread attached the victim to the crime, this would mean that the victim, through the act of forgiveness, should cut the thread between the perpetrator and the crime and then remain alone with the crime. This situation is shown in Figure 3.1.

It would be better to cut the victim from the crime. Then the perpetrator would be able to attempt to come to terms with her crime on her own, and the situation would be as shown in Figure 3.2.[15]

Anyone seeking a path of forgiveness can initially detach themselves from identifying with the crime by unambiguously associating it with the perpetrator and if necessary, in a later second step, detaching the identification between the image of the crime they have detached and the image of the perpetrator.

What we describe individually as "identity" is equivalent to what we describe socially as a "role". We can only form an image of who we are in the mirror of how we are treated and seen by other key individuals. We become the person as whom we are treated, provided that we do not veto this process by saying or thinking something along the lines of the following: "I'm not the person as whom you treat me. I'm different to how you see me." It is rarely possible for a child to lodge a veto of this kind. This calls for reflection of a sort that requires new encounters with individuals or groups who allow us to see a more helpful image of ourselves than anything offered to us by earlier attachment figures.

If I wish to say, "I'm not the person as whom you treat me," it's a good idea for me to find thoughts and words for who I am instead. This means finding internal films with images and dialogues, and with the bodily sensations and emotions of an experienced "alternative identity". This demarcation between identity on the one hand and the roles and identities offered by other individuals and groups on the other is of course important with regard to trauma, or in other words a context where we are talking about perpetrators and victims.

People are traumatised particularly often by the behaviour of their parents or other people in their family of origin. This presents a dilemma; it seems to many clients wishing to develop a positive self-image that they must renounce the people

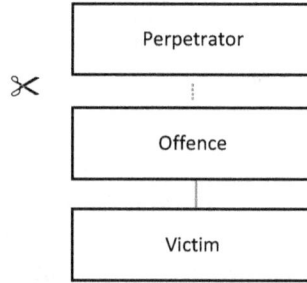

Figure 3.1 Supporting the perpetrator by asking the victim for forgiveness

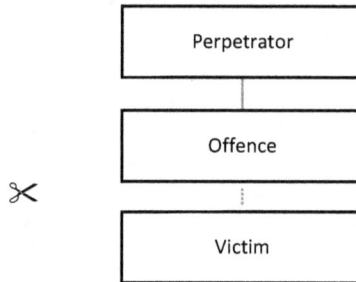

Figure 3.2 Supporting the victim by leaving the guilt with the perpetrator

who did not promote this image and who often also continue being unsupportive of it. On the other hand, these clients feel a strong need to belong to the members of their family of origin, and the role and identity offered by these latter is perceived by clients as highly plausible. Later offers of identity often appear constructed and implausible. Clients sometimes feel disloyal and guilty if they distance themselves from the interpretations of their family of origin. The same often applies in the case of religious and ideological communities with family-like structures. Who are they if not the person they regarded themselves as for so long because that is how they were regarded?

From a biological perspective, it is safe to say that humans are herd animals. In a herd there is nothing more important than belonging. An outcast from the group risks death.[16] A safe place within the system is vitally important. Yet anyone in a weak position who puts up too much resistance against the roles offered in the herd and against its leader will gain not a better position, but instead a position as an outsider or outcast from the herd.

Children who rebel against violent parents must expect more violence. A further problem is that they are typically unable to present an alternative for who they are, and certainly not one that would be accepted by the adults with the outcome of a recognised role within the family. What matters is having a place in the family. Having a place means having a role, and having a role means having an identity. In case of doubt, a child decides that it's better to have a bad role than no role at all. It's better to have an identity as an inferior person than no identity at all. Since we do not typically reinvent our identity, decisions of this kind are carried with us into our adulthood, and updated a thousand times over. It would appear that people are loathe to relinquish their childhood traumas because these latter are conceptually linked to belonging, roles, and identities. In many cases it apparently proves impossible to find a solution that allows them not only to experience belonging to their family of origin, but at the same time to live an autonomous life and be different.

How can we help people to break away from the role and identity assigned to them without losing their sense of belonging to a system of origin that is also significant for their experience of identity?

How can the identity experienced by individuals described as victims or describing themselves as victims be detached from the role assigned by the "perpetrator" and his system, without us trivialising or implicitly justifying the injustice suffered?

Once again we need to make some helpful distinctions, and we can follow the rule of "separating problems" to do so. The following distinctions have proven useful …

1. … between role assignment and identity (social noise):

"One of the basic principles of systemic therapy is as follows: 'What Hans says about Peter says a lot about Hans and nothing about Peter.'"[17]

"I once saw a slogan that said, 'Regardless of what your mummy says, you're a princess.' What do you think about that? No child is born bad, and if people think badly about the child, that's on them rather than the child."

"If you go on a photo safari and the buffalo at the waterhole grunt at you, they're not doing it because of you. They didn't invent grunting on your behalf. There are lots of different social noises: the warning grunts, territorial demarcation grunts, hierarchising grunts, mating grunts and other social noises are all different. You might notice, 'That's how grunting is done where they come from.' And when you get home, you might also realise that things are just the same there. It has nothing to do with you."[18]

2. … between experienced treatment and personal value (20-dollar note):

"How much is this 20-dollar note worth? Are you sure? Now if I crumple it up and stamp on it, what's it worth now? If I bring it to the grocery store, what is its value then? 5 dollars? 10 dollars? 15 dollars? "[19]

3. … between the judgement handed down against the accused and the accuser:

"Who ought to be ashamed? It is normally not the one who was shamed that should be ashamed, but the one who shamed him. What do you think?"[20]

4. ... between intention and implementation:

"Another basic principle is as follows: 'Parents do the best they can.'[21] That doesn't mean that what happened was the best. It might have been the worst. It simply means that your parents didn't do what they did because they wanted the bad things to happen, but because they couldn't find a better way of dealing with it. Probably because they didn't know any better. They were overstretched or wrongly informed, for example about priorities in life."

"What must he have suffered before he became someone who would do to his daughter something that no father should ever do to his daughter?"[22]

5. ... between love that was not experienced and love that did not exist:

"Even if no love has arrived, that does not always mean that no love was there. Sometimes the packages are packed with love and not sent, and sometimes they are sent and do not arrive."[23]

6. ... between belonging to the system and assent or autonomy:

"I belong to you, and I do it differently. Differently to how you did it, differently to what you thought was right, and differently to what you planned for me."

"I'll take both: I belong to you in my own way, and I'm different to how you see me. More different than you can imagine."[24]

7. ... between what is rejected and what is retained (strawberry mash and manure):

If I were to serve you up a dish of mashed strawberries with liquid manure, would you eat it? Of course not ... But if someone was holding you captive, you'd eat it in order not to starve. If children receive a mixture of violence and love, or neglect and care, they take what they get. Now imagine a machine that 'unwhisks' the mashed strawberries and liquid manure, right down to the last molecule. The strawberry mash is ejected on the left, and that stands for everything you have experienced in terms of love, respect, and the furthering and expansion of your possibilities, while the liquid manure is ejected on the right, and that corresponds to violence, neglect, lack of respect, humiliation, and the constriction of your possibilities. Once the mixture has been separated to perfection, you get handed the container with the strawberry mash, and the container with the liquid manure is handed over to a disposal company, which might convert it into heat and electricity in a methane plant.[25]

What all of these approaches have in common is that the aspects of experience associated with positively experienced belonging and self-image are retained and distinguished from the aspects associated with humiliation and threat.

Generally speaking, it should be recognised that what has happened (the crime) is not a trivial issue, that it was suffered without being deserved and that it does not contain any message about the value and nature of the suffering individual. Persons whose behaviour caused trauma to others are not exonerated with a view to what they did, but with a view to the potential they have in principle as humans, or are acknowledged for their own suffering, which is interpreted as facilitating what they did that caused suffering.

3.1.3 Crisis

We interpret who we are in the mirror of how we are interpreted and treated by the groups to which we belong.

When a close attachment figure dies, there is a shift in the interpretative framework within which people assign roles and identities to themselves and to others. This shift is associated with a search for the significance of the deceased in our own life, but also with questions about our own place in the life of the deceased, of the group, and of the world. The answers given by the surviving relative or friend to questions like these also depend on the answers given by others in the system, just like their answers depend on the answers of others.

In the same way that a flock of birds circles around in the air without any individual bird deciding on the route that should be followed, with the route instead resulting from the interaction of all of the members of the flock, there is a change in the behaviour and experience of all of a group's members if changes in the group composition require a reinterpretation of their status.

Yet that is the external perspective. The view from the inside looks different. Numbness, emotional pain, inner struggles, and confusion play a central role in what we call grief.

Grief is regularly experienced by people as a crisis of reality and identity. They describe their experiences of grief using words such as the following:

- "Everything feels so unreal."
- "I feel like I'm looking down on myself."
- "Sometimes I don't even know who I am any more."
- "It's like the ground is slipping away from under my feet."
- "Everything inside me is topsy turvy."

Those who believe that their relative has not "gone away" or been extinguished, but is still invisibly "there" and continues to live, experience grief in a less severe form.

Moving house

A geriatric nurse told me, "I'm surrounded by so many people whom I like, and so many of them die – if I were to grieve for all of them, I'd never stop grieving. Instead, I say to myself, 'They've just moved house'".

Inviting those in mourning to see the deceased not as "lost" or "gone" but as people who continue to be invisibly with them typically reduces their burden significantly. Grief work is not about accepting a loss, but about transforming the grief to the extent that the bereaved can take the deceased along with them as they live the rest of their life. This concept – which was highlighted by Roland Kachler[26] – is of central importance for successful grief counselling. In my experience, observations such as the following can deliver tremendous relief in a short space of time to those mourning the dead.

The first day of your invisible life together

> The day on which your brother died was the first day of your invisible life together. After all, he's not gone anywhere as far as you're concerned. He's there in your heart. I don't want you to continue living without your brother – I'd like you to continue living with him as an invisible companion. You can do that from a place of deep belief, or call it imagination.[27]

It can also be helpful to convey to those in mourning that what they are experiencing has a purpose, and that the internal reorganisation they are currently undergoing will lead to a positive outcome, even if they are unable to recognise that at the present time.[28]

One might wonder why grief often affects people so greatly and for so long even though this consumes enormous amounts of energy and poses a risk to health as a result. A possible answer is that people unconsciously subscribe to the idea that, "the greater the pain, the greater the love", or in other words that the values associated with grief are unconsciously linked with the expression of symptoms.

Separating the symptoms that are experienced from the values associated with them to date[29] has proven very successful in situations of grief and separation.

Break-ups of relationships and families are sometimes even harder to cope with than bereavements for the individuals involved. This is firstly because there is often a long period of back and forth between hope and disappointment, and secondly because the other's behaviour is assigned a meaning in terms of the individual's own identity. If a relationship becomes unstable, the relevant interpretations of identity – the individual's own identity and the other's identity – also become unstable. The other person appears no longer to be the person the individual thought he was for many years; what is more, the individual often no longer recognises himself and is interpreted by others as having undergone a change in personality.

Since we need dependability in our interpretation of ourselves and our interpretation of the world, these fluctuations in our models of roles and identities are supremely stressful.

These dynamics become even more complicated in love triangles as well as in families where children or other important relatives switch sides or come down in favour of an unexpected side.

An intervention to reduce suffering in a love triangle or following a break-up can be found under the heading "Dividing up the ex-husband".[30]

Bullying can be experienced by the bullied as a splitting of identity where the internal self cannot decide which experience of identity should primarily be experienced – a more attractive identity put forward by fewer people or by people who are not currently present, or an identity that is put forward by people who are powerful (in terms of influence, rank, or number) but who assign to the bullied a negative role and devalue him. What effect does that have on a human's experience of identity?

In terms of how he handles the situation, it is of decisive importance whether he succeeds in continuing to see the people who previously surrounded him as his primary reference group when determining who he is, or whether he involuntarily prefers to use those who now surround him as a basis for his self-interpretation. This may be the case because the people who now surround him can be seen and heard in the present moment, and the impression of the way in which they treat him is constantly being refreshed and corroborated by new impressions, whereas the memories of earlier attachment figures may have faded.

People in barracks or custody who are isolated from their attachment figures can find themselves facing similar challenges. Solitary confinement is often referred to as a form of torture. This is attributable firstly to the fact that belonging is such a primeval basic need that a loud internal alarm is sounded if we do not experience belonging for a long and indefinite period, and secondly to the fact that the prisoner's experience of identity may disintegrate if the memories of the group to which he belongs fade.

The need for belonging becomes yet stronger if the individual is subject to powerlessness and isolation – so strong that it is relatively easy for prisoners in isolation to reach a point where they declare their solidarity with those keeping them imprisoned and come to share their views (Stockholm syndrome, brainwashing, self-denunciation).

Changed allegiances can result in a changed experience of identity within days or weeks, with corresponding changes in worldview and social behaviour.

3.1.4 New allegiances

Therapists are generally trusted to be experts on matters of personality. The authority assigned to them in this connection is exceptionally useful when offering clients options for helpfully reinterpreting themselves and their position within their family of origin and among their current reference persons in family and work settings.

Generally speaking, it is a good idea for the client herself, through therapy, to reach a new self-interpretation – of her gifts and opportunities, of the way in which her behaviour and experience should be evaluated, of her potential, her role in the structure of other key figures, and of what otherwise characterises her as a personality. A new self-image of this kind will only be accepted by the client if it is vivid, relevant, and plausible for her.[31]

With his professional authority, positive attention and resource-oriented attitude, the therapist can thus become the guarantor of a new experience of role and identity for the client.

In order to identify options for new and helpful roles and identities so that the client can locate herself positively in the orbit of other important people (her "herd"), use can be made of helpful people from earlier or now, ancestors, possible or fictitious persons, or resourceful "parts" of the client.[32] If the client reorganises the internally experienced arrangement of her "home and herd", her implicit verbal and non-verbal communications will involuntarily transmit other options for positioning her within a structure of roles to the important persons in her environment, meaning that this structure may start to shift.

The good mother in you – out of you – for you

A seminar attendee who had achieved great things in her career advocated for others who needed or might need her help, in a supremely caring and committed manner. She herself accepted hardly any help from them. She seemed to me to be proud of giving more than she took. I said to her, "You know that I hugely admire your skill and the way you help others. On the other hand, it could also be said that you like giving to others and dislike taking from others because you'd like to be absolutely certain that your give-and-take account is not in the red, or in other words that no one can demand anything from you because they once gave you something, and perhaps even demand more than they got from you. Perhaps you once had a bad experience when you accepted something from someone else, and later they demanded something back from you. What do you think?" The woman answered, with tears in her eyes, "I've never thought about it like that before, but I believe you're right."

"Imagine the person you are who can be very, very kind, like a best friend or big sister or a very loving mother, and imagine that this person steps out of you, crouches down in front of you and looks you very warmly and lovingly in the eyes, and asks you to accept from her warmth and understanding, solidarity, respect, and every other kind of loving acknowledgement – would you be able to accept it from her? It might be easier to accept it from her because she's just a version of you, after all, and if you ever needed to give her something back, for starters you'd know – because you know her – that she isn't demanding it, and also that if you did ever want to give her something back, you'd ultimately be giving it to yourself. If she gives you the warmth and respect and recognition that you do not accept from others, is that OK?"

"Yes, that's OK with me," she agreed, visibly moved. She later told me that this encounter had been very helpful for her, and had set a lot in motion internally.

An intervention of this kind initially alters the woman's attitude to herself; it then influences her ability to accept care from others, and then her opportunities to advocate for others and give them gifts, which again has an impact on the willingness of the others to receive gifts from her (and perhaps from others). The people surrounding the client will strike a new balance in their roles towards her, which will in turn influence their relationships amongst each other. Which of her friends will now develop a particularly warm or relaxed or committed relationship with her? A change in one relationship in the system (including a relationship with one-self) leads to shifts in all the relevant relationships.

Who an individual regards himself as being is based on the people to whom he feels like he belongs, with whom he has solidarity and whose values he shares, and the people of whom he is critical and whose values he condemns. It results from his position in the sphere of the key others he sees himself as being surrounded by in his imagination or in his current situation. *An individual sees himself in the way that he has learned that others see and treat him.* This is true unless he distances himself from the others who are assigning roles, thereby expressing the following idea: I am not who *you* see me as; I am who the *others* (for example my grandparents, my friends, my therapist) see me as.

A systematic reassessment of what has previously been experienced from the perspective of new prioritisations of values allows a person to feel a sense of belonging to those who adhere to *these* values, and to experience himself as one of them. Trying to devalue or erase the memory of people who on the one hand contributed to the trauma and on the other hand, as parental attachment figures, also offered orientation in life, offers less chance of success, however. It is a better idea to keep everything that is worth keeping, perhaps all the more so if there's not much of it, and to reject what is to be rejected. A comprehensive sorting of biographical memories along these lines is impossible at the level of conscious thought. But who knows what the unconscious is capable of?

In the case of clients with early and extensive intrafamilial traumas (often associated with a borderline personality disorder (BPD) diagnosis), the intervention "Strawberry mash and manure"[33] has delivered positive outcomes. It involves drawing a boundary (between what the client accepts for herself as appropriate treatment and what she rejects as inappropriate) not along the line between acceptance or rejection of a parent, but perpendicular to this line. An involuntary distinction is thus imposed between behaviours that have strengthened her and those that have weakened her. The decision about where exactly this line should run is removed from conscious thought and memory, and assigned to a competent unconscious authority.

Similarly, the client can be invited to reorder needs for autonomy and a sense of belonging to parents and other attachment figures by recognising her own decision as a characteristic of belonging instead of the behaviour alleged to be good in the past. The following intervention can help clients to orient themselves in a new experience of roles and identities.

I'll take both (autonomy and belonging)

The client can be invited to say the following to her parents: "I'll take both: I belong to you and I'm doing it differently – differently to how you did it, and also differently to how you thought that I should do it." By saying this, the client separates two concepts that were previously merged, and tells the parents from her head to do the same. She makes a distinction between belonging to the family of origin and the behaviour expected there (or her autonomy), and thus between the value she feels that she has as a person and specific values held by the family.[34]

Back in Chapter 2, we discussed the changes that are possible if a person experienced by the client as traumatising is removed (in the client's imagination) from the client's head and sent to receive instruction in a "heavenly university of love and wisdom" until the client perceives some form of purification in that person, an exposing of his potential and perhaps a trace of enlightenment.[35]

Subject to the proviso that the suffering that has been experienced must be recognised and not trivialised, the far-reaching effect of such an intervention is that clients – in order to modify the agonising memories that are experienced as timeless and currently present – develop a better relationship with the "father in their head" (or the relevant person). To date, the latter had made a negative contribution to the client's perspective and self-perspective within the framework of roles in her environment. This contribution is now corrected in some sense, meaning that it offers the client an improved role and identity. The client's altered relationship with the transformed attachment figure also generates altered relationships ...

- with herself,
- with the relevant person (if they are still alive) as a physically real person,
- with other attachment figures (e.g. her mother), and
- between these attachment figures.

The following is of course a valid question in this connection: what happens if the physical person who was the source of the trauma continues to offer degrading roles to the client? Might this lead to the collapse of any positive therapeutic outcome that has been achieved, perhaps temporarily?

Experience tends to show that interventions that alter the client's image of the person who has behaved in such a way as to inflict stress also tend to reduce suffering even if that person does not fundamentally desist from their behaviour.

As a basic principle, we must take care not to offer only interventions such as those outlined above in cases where humiliation and abuse is ongoing. Not everyone behaves appropriately after being examined and treated respectfully by a counterpart. Yet even Jesus' tenet of loving your enemy was based not on the idea that being nice changes opponents into friends, but rather on the concept of preserving one's own dignity and challenging the other and his behaviour by choosing not to mirror his derogatory behaviour, but instead reversing it.[36]

It is better in this case to take people out of the zone of suffering wherever possible, for example through sick leave or job moves for people suffering excessively as a result of their working conditions. In other cases, it might prove successful to immunise people to a high degree against their suffering in the situation by "de-emotionalising" it.

3.2 Abandonment and trauma

It is in relationships that we are hurt, and it is in relationships that we are healed.

That also means that not all of our conventional therapeutic arrangements are a good way of generating healing experiences. Some are probably not particularly good for anyone, and some are unsuitable for certain cultures, certain individuals, or certain family set-ups. Every course of therapy must be adapted to the needs and habits of the clients to whom it is provided.

A Rwandan once talked about his tribe's experiences with psychotherapy:

> You know, we had a lot of trouble with Western mental health workers who came here immediately after the genocide, and we had to ask some of them to leave ... Their practice did not involve being outside in the sun, like you're describing, which is, after all, where you begin to feel better. There was no music or drumming to get your blood flowing again. There was no sense that everyone had taken the day off so that the entire community could come together to try to lift you up and bring you back to joy. There was no acknowledgment that the depression is something invasive and external that could actually be cast out of you again ... Instead, they would take people one at a time into these dingy little rooms and have them sit around for an hour or so and talk about bad things that had happened to them. We had to get them to leave the country.[37]

What we call trauma is associated with the perceived loss of safety and belonging, with the disappearance of a place (or a good place) in society or of an emotionally and mentally secure existence, with loneliness, and also with a loss of control over one's own safe space and with the loss of one's home country. The experience of being defencelessly exposed to a danger contributes to the traumatic potential of a situation, as does the feeling that the source of the danger cannot be clearly located, or that the evolution of a dangerous situation cannot be gauged.[38]

According to the French neuropsychiatrist Boris Cyrulnik, soldiers who had 30 seconds to get themselves to safety in response to a siren because their camp was under fire by rockets suffered an enormous rate of traumatisation, despite the fact that almost none of them died or were injured. The rate was significantly higher than during deployments involving contact with the enemy because the soldiers experienced themselves not as "masters of the events", but as objects at which the rockets were being shot.[39]

Cyrulnik states that soldiers about to embark on a dangerous deployment were asked beforehand to write a letter to their loved ones at home, to place it in an envelope, and to wait until after the deployment to decide whether to send it or to do something else with it. Symptoms of PTSD were almost never identified in the relevant soldiers. The rate of traumatisation among these soldiers was in fact lower than among those who remained in the camp.[40] Cyrulnik believes that this effect can be explained by the fact that when writing their letters, the soldiers oriented themselves internally towards a familiar, close human relationship representing a situation where they had control over their life. The soldiers who remained in the camp were focused on events in which they did not experience themselves as playing a structuring role. In my opinion, the soldiers who took part in the experiment simulated an experience of home and of safety in belonging. The fact that they did not send the letter before the deployment ensured that this experience persisted as a framework within which the experience of danger was anchored. In the context of war-induced trauma, Cyrulnik refers to the stress involved in experiencing oneself as an object to which something is done. Particularly profound forms of trauma result from humiliation by others who gain a subjective benefit from their treatment of others like non-humans (animals, plants, objects, or simply nothing at all). The individual who suffers this humiliation – typically in social isolation – must fight against the role as a non-human becoming his identity. His challenge is to resist the identity that is presented to him as something without any alternative, even though there is no one present who can reflect and confirm his humanity to him. This also includes the disconcerting experience of being treated "like dirt" by others who ignore our verbal questions and contributions. If we experience ourselves as part of a system which frequently treats us in that way, we must resist the temptation to treat ourselves as non-existent.

Trauma creates paralysis: paralysis of the muscles, the circulation, the voice, the ability to breathe freely, the senses; for example bodily sensations, spatial hearing, the regulation of brightness, emotions, thoughts, and many other bodily functions. *What releases paralysis resolves trauma.*

3.2.1 Origins

Generally speaking, we call experiences traumatic if they involve a person being exposed in a defenceless state to an overwhelming threat that is associated with fear and horror, and sometimes also disgust. The individual experiences what is happening to him while lacking the power to do anything about it. The term "trauma" is used if the associated physical, mental, and social defence reactions do not recede by themselves, but instead persist.

Witnesses of events of this kind may also be traumatised if they identify with the person who suffered harm to the extent that they themselves feel affected.

If we ask people who come to therapy, "How long have you felt this stress, and what else was happening at the time?", they almost always – regardless of whether the symptoms are mental or physical – talk about times of particular stress. If they tell us about interpersonal conflicts and if we ask, "Can you remember previous times in your life when you behaved in a similar way or experienced a similar emotional state?", they very often explain that these things have been happening to them since childhood.

If we thus trace back to its earliest detectable preliminary stages the history of their burdens (such as depression, mania, psychosis, addiction, compulsion and anxiety-related problems), we encounter experiences of "alarmed loneliness" almost without exception. The spectrum of these experiences encompasses in particular …

- physical isolation (*incubator, internment, imprisonment*),
- loss of close attachment figures (*bereavements, separation, giving away children*),
- risk of death at an early age (*acute or chronic, including as a foetus*),

- emotional isolation (*depression and grief of relatives, including as a foetus*),
- social or physical neglect,
- feeling unwelcome,
- violence and humiliation by attachment figures,
- orchestration of intractable moral conflicts by attachment figures.

Some people think of a stressful individual event when they hear the word "trauma", but often the biographical and social circumstances in which such an event is processed are of more decisive importance than what actually happens. This explains why the same event is hugely harmful for *one* person and not harmful at all for *another.*

As I see it, the traumatic potential of a situation does not necessarily depend on the actual level of danger, but is essentially determined by three factors:

- the level of chronically experienced isolation and defencelessness (i.e. loneliness, neglect, or emotional isolation),
- the subjective intensity of the threat (highly plausible threatening fantasies can thus also have a traumatising effect),
- the proportion of the client's lifetime for which the threat has been present (early stresses as well as long-lasting or frequent stresses are particularly problematic).

When considering the proportion of a lifetime for which a threat has been experienced, attention should be paid not only to the client's age at a particular moment in time, but also to issues such as how long and how often the client has been affected by similar stresses that are potentially triggered in the current situation.

Trauma is organised in series. If we go forwards along the timeline of an individual's biography (or in other words from the original events to the therapy session), this means that the earlier, the more intensely, and the more often a person is exposed to stressful events such as those referred to at the beginning, the more likely it is that he will react to later associated events with an increased level of alertness and process them traumatically. This implies that people who have experienced early traumas typically accumulate far more traumatically processed experiences in the course of their later biography than others who have grown up within a protected framework from the outset. The numbers on the following diagram firstly designate the sequence of the stressful events, but also express an aspect of the potential to cause stress of the respective event: the lower the number, the greater the potential impacts of the event. In other words, the earlier in life traumatic situations occur, the more problems may result as a consequence of them.

Observations from therapeutic work indicate that people who experienced significant stresses as foetuses (accidents, attempted abortions, maternal depression or severe grief, death of a twin) often react in a comparable way to people who were traumatised as an infant. There are simply fewer opportunities for a foetus to be traumatised in this respect, since he does not perceive threats via the eyes and ears, and only in a limited manner via the surface of his body.

It Is clear that early and frequent traumas typically result in higher concentrations of later events that are processed traumatically. Since therapy typically looks backwards from the current stresses towards the preceding events, this has the following implication.

Whenever people exhibit defensive reactions that are much more powerful than appears to be explicable on the basis of the situation, it is worth asking about the background. "It's understandable that you'd find that stressful. Which of your previous experiences might have meant that it is even more unpleasant for you than for certain other people? Have you perhaps experienced something approximately similar before?" It is often the case that we are then told about the seventh, sixth, or fifth events, or perhaps even the first event straight away. And naturally we can also cut right to the chase, as follows: "Did anything out of the ordinary happen at the very start of your life?" The therapist then often gets to hear about "Episode 1", which is a major help in structuring further work (Figure 3.3).

For example, I asked a young man: "How long have you been afraid of spiders?" "For a very long time, ever since I was a child." "Do you remember the first time you were afraid of a spider?" "I don't know whether it was the first time, but I remember digging a hole in the ground with a small stick. Suddenly a spider popped out of nowhere and attacked me – or at least that was how it seemed to me as a child." "How old were you at the time?" "Three." "Was there anything special going on at that point in your life?" "My parents separated when I was three."

However, what is also remarkable is the fact that certain children (and then the same individuals once they reach adulthood) exhibit trauma-related reactions for which no direct triggering event in the child's life can be identified, yet a stress that easily explains this behaviour by the child is all the more obvious in the life of a parent (or sometimes even in the life of a grandparent). In this instance, the child's history of trauma appears to be the continuation of a series of traumas in the family's history (Figure 3.4).

As explained above, smaller numbers stand for earlier events and thus for situations that have a stress potential which is in principle higher. My impression is that stresses from a family's past history have a greater impact if their effect extends over several generations than if they affect only one parent.

This raises fundamental questions. For example:

Is it possible for a child to exhibit a claustrophobic reaction because his father was buried alive under rubble for several days during the war?

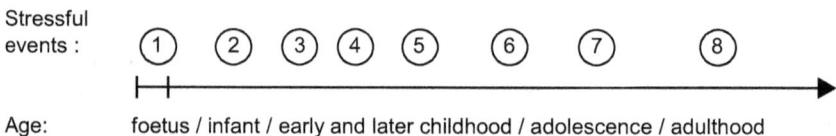

Stressful events : ① ② ③ ④ ⑤ ⑥ ⑦ ⑧

Age: foetus / infant / early and later childhood / adolescence / adulthood

Figure 3.3 Trauma organised in series within a person's biography

Stressful
events:

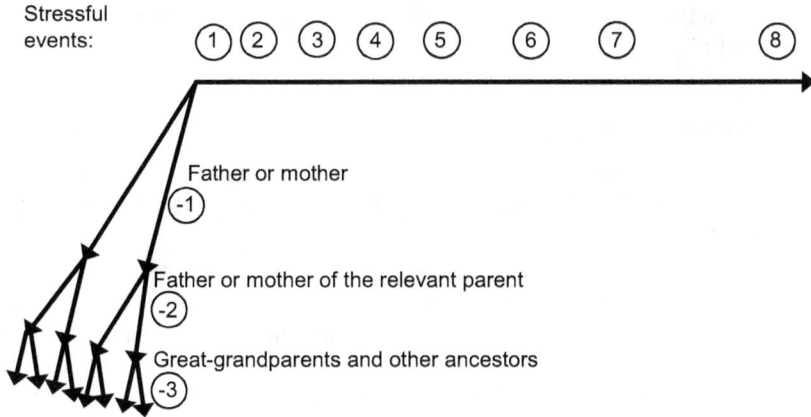

Figure 3.4 Trauma organised in series within a family biography

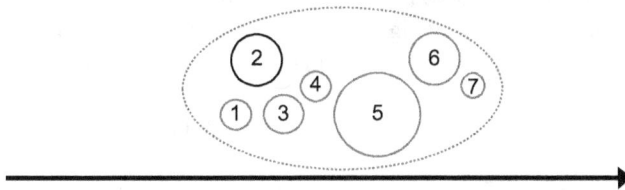

Figure 3.5 Trauma organised in a cluster of events

Can a child develop an eating disorder because her mother came close to dying from starvation as a young woman?

Can a person become suicidal because several family members completed suicide before his birth, even though the family never speaks about the circumstances of their deaths?

Perhaps it is the case that phenomena of these kind – which can certainly be observed very often – might be explained in the future through epigenetic or other mechanisms for storing information from previous generations. Or perhaps information might also be encoded in the overall behaviour of a family or group, and this information can be decoded by an individual's unconscious.

Trauma is organised in clusters. If several stressful events occur in close chronological succession, the stresses associated with them accumulate. The cluster of events can be regarded as an integrated whole. A small additional stress that is more symbolic than significant may ultimately be enough to cause a breakdown (Figure 3.5).

I once asked a woman who came to therapy with the symptoms of a major depressive episode the following question: "Was your depression triggered by anything?" She talked about difficulties with her mother and her daughter. "In the end, all it took was for a customer to say to me, 'I'm just not keen on what you're offering me,' and I broke down."[41]

3.2.2 Triggers

In simplified terms, one can distinguish between a traumatic original situation (or chains and clouds of such situations and the stimuli that trigger trauma-related behaviour).

Anything that was experienced as characteristic of the situation, either during the original stress or in rapid chronological succession, may become a triggering stimulus. Such stimuli may include aspects of the dangerous situation (the bank robber's hair colour) or relatively arbitrary stimuli that were experienced at more or less the same time as the original event and can symbolise a danger (the motorway on which the hostage drove home after being freed). Triggering stimuli can be very specific (spiders) or quite generalised (the space outside the apartment), or there may be a specific combination of stimuli. For example, a woman who had been thrown from a galloping horse developed a phobia that meant that she could no longer walk over bridges. A swinging suspension bridge proved particularly challenging. The stimuli that were combined in this instance were height *and* instability *and* movement.

Triggering stimuli may be perceived via any sensory channel:

- acoustic *(New Year's fireworks for a traumatised war veteran),*
- optical *(bank buildings for the bank robber's hostage),*
- kinaesthetic *(the head being touched following a fall resulting in head injuries),*
- olfactory *(a fragrance similar to that worn by the rapist),*
- gustatory *(honey after being forced to try some as a child),*
- immunological *(pollen that was in the air during the original event).*

It was pointed out above that trauma is organised in chains, and that trauma is organised in clouds. It might be the case that there are a series of consecutive original events giving rise to different stimuli that trigger phobias in each instance.

For example, a client might have developed a motorway phobia after spending a long time in a traffic jam. When asked by her therapist if she could think of any reasons why the experience with the traffic jam might have had such a major impact, she might say firstly that her husband had just left her, and secondly that she had already developed a phobia of lifts by that point, after being trapped in one for several hours. In any case, she had "always" suffered from claustrophobia to some extent.

The therapist might respond, "Always? Since your birth? What was going on back then?" The woman might answer that she got trapped in the birth canal and was pulled out using a ventouse. Afterwards she had spent several days under observation in the Neonatal Intensive Care Unit (NICU) due to oxygen deprivation.

The therapist can then follow up by asking, "Did any of your parents or grand-parents suffer from claustrophobia or anything similar?" The woman might answer that her father had in fact struggled with claustrophobia after being buried alive under rubble during the war, when he was a young man, and only being dug out again after a couple of days.

Although it might appear that enough potential reasons for the emergence of the client's symptoms have been identified, it is sometimes worth continuing to ask whether there were any events in the life of the mother or the grandparents that are associated with fear, confinement, or suffocation.

It thus seems to be the case that the woman has exhibited claustrophobic behaviour since her birth, that she has developed a phobia of lifts and other enclosed moving vehicles (cars, trains, planes) since the experience with the lift, and additionally a phobia of driving on motorways since the experience with the traffic jam.

It might furthermore be the case that she has had asthmatic tendencies since being deprived of oxygen during birth, and that these tendencies were reinforced during the experiences in the lift and on the motorway.

She might also have started to have nightmares since the experience on the motorway, as well as becoming prone to sleep apnoea.

3.2.3 Effects

The impacts of traumas become noticeable if they result in mentally or physically associated over- or underreactions that restrict the well-being and possibilities for action of the affected individuals themselves and of the other people in their surroundings.

A distinction should be made between direct reactions by the client to traumatic triggers, complex chronic reactions (syndromes, mental and physical illnesses) and impacts that result from interactions with other people or larger systems (conflicts).

One might ask whether the symptoms listed below as examples are "always" to be explained as being rooted in trauma. In systemic work, "always is always wrong". The following are examples of symptoms that are observed with conspicuously high frequency as reactions to traumatic stimuli.

Examples of reactions that tend to be mentally connoted are as follows:

- paralysis,
- hesitant thinking and speaking,
- emotional numbness,
- experience of helplessness and powerlessness,
- confusion,
- panic,
- anger and aggressive impulses (shouting, hitting),
- disgust,
- absences (trance states, sometimes with unresponsiveness),
- uncontrollable, inadequate-seeming crying,

and, experienced more chronically:

- episodes of depression,
- episodes of mania,
- episodes of psychosis,
- episodes of addiction,
- self-harming behaviour,
- eating disorders,
- sleep disorders,
- sexual disorders,

and many more.

Examples of reactions that tend to be physically connoted are as follows:

- spasms,
- nausea,
- headaches and sore throats,
- physical numbness,
- itching,
- palpitations, circulatory disorders,
- shortness of breath, flat, or laboured breathing,
- strained, jangling, or cracking voice,
- temporary visual impairment,
- dizziness and impaired balance,
- loss of consciousness,
- epileptic conditions,

and, experienced more chronically:

- autoimmune diseases (allergies, asthma, Crohn's disease),
- inflammatory diseases (tonsilitis, cystitis),
- fibromyalgia,
- high blood pressure,
- migraines,
- tinnitus,
- tension (bruxism, torticollis, lumbago),

and many more.

From the perspective of an observer, a distinction can be made between triggers that appear trivial and harmless to others (moths, the sound of people eating) and triggers that might cause understandable concern in others, but are not expected to lead to extreme reactions (police officers, dogs). Similarly, a distinction can be made between reactions that are significantly stronger than the reaction expected or that differ from the reaction expected.

A recurring behavioural reaction is almost certainly co-generated by trauma if it is many times stronger than would be expected on the basis of normal interpersonal contacts. The same is true if the nature of the reaction rather than its strength is completely out of sync with the situation.

Hypo-agitated reactions such as the following are also frequent but less conspicuous in interpersonal contacts:

- paralysis,
- sluggishness and lack of energy,
- excessive yawning (yawn syndrome),
- excessive tendency to diminutivise (Bambi syndrome),
- anticipatory self-retraction and self-subjugation,
- strong emphasis on being kind,
- physical numbness,
- lack of emotions,
- shyness with mute self-abasement,
- withdrawal,
- accommodation of others' needs without regard for any personal disadvantages suffered,
- avoidant behaviour.

It is possible to observe in kindergartens and school classes, and in the field of child and adolescent psychiatry, that girls tend to display hypo-agitated forms of traumatic reaction, while boys tend to act out traumatic reactions in a clearly visible and audible manner. The fact that significantly more boys than girls are diagnosed with attention-deficit hyperactivity disorder (ADHD) may be attributable in part to the fact that the effects of trauma are often confused with those of ADHD in boys, and in part to the fact that any traumas they suffer may exacerbate their ADHD-related behaviours.

Relationship problems are almost always caused or jointly caused by trauma, because the level of stress experienced by one partner as a result of the other's behaviour depends to a significant extent on the stresses suffered previously as a result of comparable behaviours displayed by caregivers in childhood (or behaviours that appeared similar from an external perspective). Behaviours of this kind generate particularly strong or abnormal protective reactions, which often generate a stress reaction in the other partner. A spiral of retraumatisation results for both partners. In the context of traumatic stress, the mutual contingency (circularity) of human behaviour creates a problem. Generally speaking, it is not necessarily the successful interactions that are stabilised in relationships, but those that are likely to produce each other reciprocally in a circular fashion.[42]

Perhaps one partner is alarmed at the other's withdrawn, distrustful-seeming behaviour because he is involuntarily reminded of unpleasant episodes from his childhood. He responds irritably and impatiently. The other feels alarmed by this, perhaps because she in turn remembers unpleasant scenes from her past. She reacts with paralysis and withdrawal. This alarms her partner, who becomes even louder, based on the principle that "more is better". The other feels even more alarmed and becomes even more withdrawn and tense. This is how loops of mutual retraumatisation are created. Each of the two partners will believe that their behaviour was merely a reaction to what the other was doing, and each will believe that they are merely protecting themselves.

3.2.4 Resolution

A trauma is healed if the individual can both recall the original situation and perceive the triggering stimuli without this resulting in underactive or overactive physiological states (paralysis, immobility, numbness, depression or panic, violent bouts of temper, fits of crying, manic-euphoric states).

Things can get a little more complicated than that, however. Let's return our attention to the hypothetical case of the woman with a phobia of driving on motorways. This phobia had developed in stages, and so in fact the woman was suffering not from a single fear, but from a variety of fears.

If the client's mission is to work together with the therapist to resolve the motorway phobia, this can certainly be achieved with suitable means.[43] The therapist can enquire how long the client has been experiencing the problem, which stresses were present back when it first started, what the client thinks might have caused the problem to emerge, and whether there were any preliminary stages leading up to the current experience, perhaps in childhood or in the family's previous history. He can ask the client whether she would be happy to work on other triggering stimuli dating back to an earlier point in time (for example the lift phobia in our example); such a suggestion is typically welcomed by clients.

Both can then work on the woman's lift phobia or her experience in the lift until the client looks and sounds calm and relaxed when imagining a journey in a lift.

The therapist might issue the following invitation to the client: "Imagine the newborn you were back then, who spent so long stuck in the birth canal and was perhaps starting to turn blue – imagine taking that newborn out of you, and placing her lovingly on the armchair over there." If the client takes increasingly deep breaths and relaxes her muscles jerkily, it is likely that her birth experience left behind in her chronic tenseness, and that it is worth working further on this issue.

If the therapist asks the client to imagine her mother being called into the room and taking the newborn to her breast, and then asks the client how the baby's expression changes, her muscles and breathing will become even freer and more relaxed, mirroring the movements and breathing of the imagined child.

If no original events are identified, the therapist can also invite the client to imagine events that might have triggered or exacerbated the mentally and physically defined symptoms up until now. If the client's physiological response to this is only slight, for example as might be expected in the case of a person without this previous history, it is likely that the traumatic experience and behaviour has been resolved.

There is a good chance that the asthma and the sleep apnoea will also have been resolved, either entirely or at least for the most part. It is often helpful to create an expectation that the physical stresses might also be overcome at the same time as the mental ones; if necessary, however, attention should also be paid separately to the symptoms that are expressed physically. As ever, it is beneficial to generate plausibility in every conceivable manner for this therapeutic outcome, and to deconstruct any objections to it, or in other words remove the basis for the plausibility of these objections.

Matryoshka dolls

Are you familiar with the matryoshka dolls that come from Russia? The ones where you open up the outer doll and find a second doll inside? And then a third inside that one, a fourth, a fifth and so on? That's how I imagine therapy. We work on one problem, and while this is being resolved or after it has been resolved, a second one pops up behind it. Then we work on that, and behind that pops up a third. Sometimes we order problems according to their urgency; for example, we might be working on a case of tinnitus, and the loudest sounds disappear, but some quieter sounds are still present, and when they disappear, even quieter sounds appear, which the individual in question wouldn't even have noticed at the start. And sometimes we order problems according to their cause. We might work on depression, and when the client no longer feels paralysed, grief appears, and once the client has realised that the pain of grief does not need to be so overwhelming, shame appears, and as soon as we hand the shame back to the person who originally did the shaming, anger appears. And then while we're deciding what to do with the anger, a physical symptom appears, and when this has gone away, another appears, and finally the tears come along – tears of relief and leaving something behind ... I've observed that the problems that emerge during this process either become less and less significant or get closer and closer to the root causes, and that progress is made if there is still something that requires work. It's important to know that this is a process, and that you can start to feel better even if not everything is perfect yet.[44]

This metaphor can be used to reassure clients that progress is being made even if every stressful memory reveals another, and every disturbing emotion or bodily reaction in the course of therapy seems to be followed by another. This is often important in the case of clients that appear very disheartened (depressed) or diligent (perfectionist or compulsive), in order to build positive expectations that can lead to positive experiences.[45]

3.3 Ambivalence and conflict

Not every ambivalence is experienced as distressing. Some ambivalences can also be fun, like in the following line from a song by the pop singer Nina Hagen: "I just can't decide, everything is so nice and colourful here!"[46] An ambivalence that prompts someone to go to therapy is, however, mostly described as a problem.

From the perspective of the individual talking about it, a problem is a discrepancy between what is and what should be.

> Such discrepancies are constructed in response to phenomena that are defined as different and contradictory, for example … perceptions, wishes, opinions, behaviours and interests within a system of relationships … [which] are negatively assessed by those involved – as not belonging to the system, as diseased and evil … A solution is generated if the discrepancy between what is and what should be is resolved in the experience and behaviour of the persons perceiving the problem. This can happen if the assessment of "what is" becomes more positive, and/ or "what should be" differs less drastically from "what is", and/or the nature of the solutions that have been attempted to date is altered in such a way that the latter dispel the unwanted discrepancy between what is and what should be.[47]

Let us assume there are good reasons for both, or in other words reasons that are comprehensible if sufficient information is made available to us and that are worthy of respect. There are reasons why the situation is what it is (and previously became what it became) and why the client wishes it to be different to what it currently is. We can then take the view that every problem reported by the client is also an ambivalence, a conflict, or a double bind. The client (or the system issuing the order) appears rigid or caught in a pendulum motion between the understandable desire to hold on to the past and the equally understandable quest for something different and something new. The therapist can respectfully mirror this ambivalence (pacing), or in other words offer a therapeutic double bind:

> In systems therapy and hypnotherapy, a balance between what is and what should be [is] always a topic of discussion. If something is not right in the patient's opinion, or in other words gives rise to a need for therapy – for example chronic and disabling pain – the therapist can immediately give the pain signal positive connotations (diagnostic question: what does the pain probably want to say?), then explain how the body and its nervous system normally functions (education), and then, by means of individually tailored therapeutic strategies, encourage the overall system of the human to "drift" in the direction of his personal normality. All three tasks are inextricably linked with each other and form … a single unit.[48]

3.3.1 Problems as ambivalences

It is likely that all of the symptoms and stresses that a client presents in a therapy session can be viewed from the perspective of an ambivalence: one side of the client wants to be rid of the problem, which is why she has come to therapy. Another side doesn't want to be rid of the problem at the price she would apparently have to pay in order to lead another life, since the problem would not otherwise exist in this form.

Gunther Schmidt describes this tension as a dualism between the experience of different authorities within the personality:

> experience-related processes which ... are perceived as painful problems are ... all characterised by the fact that in the case of the relevant individuals, a conscious and voluntary "experiencing authority" desires a particular experience (e.g. well-being, joy, safety, etc.), but involuntary physical and mental processes differ materially from this experience and yet are experienced much more strongly than the former, with the result that the ego effectively feels like a victim at the mercy of these processes. Massive incongruences ... are experienced between different yet synchronous subdomains of the mental process.[49]

In this case, ambivalence does not mean being consciously torn between two things, but instead a divergence between the experiences of different internal authorities. It involves finding a good solution in an internal conflict between different strivings for safety and well-being.

If we create models of conflicts, it is important to remember that reality is largely or wholly – a point that is still open to debate among philosophers – constructed and not analysed, or in other words that "the map is not the landscape" and an image of a person is not the person that it depicts.

Internal conflicts can be represented in the following paradigmatic manner:

A) The known solutions that involve change come at too high a price.
B) Changing nothing is also unacceptable.

The situation results in, e.g. disorientation or confusion.

A) Absolute priority is given to protecting oneself against the recurrence of a traumatic situation.
B) It would be nice to lead a life without avoidance, not least because the threat is no longer present.

The situation results in, e.g. phobias or allergies.

A) One part wishes to encourage reliable relationships (loyalty, longevity).
B) Another part (mental pain) wishes to warn against the risks of loneliness.

The situation results in, e.g. long-enduring grief.

A) One part wants *one* value (comfort or pleasure in the form of chocolate).
B) Another part wants a *different* value (beauty, health).

The situation results in, e.g. addiction.

A) One part wants to send out alarm signals in the form of pain.
B) Another part finds that too unpleasant and produces paralysis and numbness.

The situation results in, e.g. depression, blackouts, or neuropathy.
Schmidt describes ambivalences of this kind in the following way:

> Even if they [clients] consciously want change (and in any case have typically
> also tried to change intentionally), they at the same time identify deeply with
> their painful reality, particularly on an unconscious, involuntary level. This can
> rapidly develop into a challenging dilemma for therapists and counsellors. After
> all, cooperation ... presupposes that we "meet" clients in their respective way
> of seeing and experiencing the world, with respect and acceptance ... If pacing
> alone were offered, therapists and counsellors would not be able to accomplish
> the task of presenting differences to the previous reality, since this reality is after
> all challenged as a result. Yet if they present differences that are intended to be
> useful, they might trigger resistance that jeopardises cooperation ... On the one
> hand, they should support and value clients' experience in a spirit of empathy
> and confirmation. On the other hand, they should present interventions that lead
> to change ... In the process they should act as experts, but never dictate what is
> good for clients and which steps they should choose.[50]

This balanced attitude towards dealing with the client's ambivalences that are
experienced consciously or unconsciously was discussed above, using the metaphor of a bridge between the problem experience and the solution experience.[51] It
plays a particular role in addressing the client's potential concerns and objections
("scepticism") to the effectiveness and sustainability of therapy,[52] the interventions
for handling objections,[53] "Corridor" and "Four quadrants", "Tetralemma", and
"Six rods".[54]

It is also an important factor in successful therapy for symptoms such as emotional or physical paralysis or numbness, which on the one hand are highly unpleasant, and on the other hand may serve the role of temporarily preventing even more
unpleasant symptoms, thereby avoiding emotional or physical overload.

3.3.2 The ambivalence of pain and numbness

Most mentally associated difficulties can be interpreted as reactions to psychological pain, in particular the pain experienced by those suffering from loneliness. As
explained, we need other people as a mirror reflecting an image of who we are.
Emotional isolation, particularly in early childhood, is a key factor in the development of traumatic experiences.[55] This results in dissociated, paralysed, or "stuck"
emotions, or emotions that have shifted from the sphere of mental experience to

that of physical experience. Many psychological stresses, and also certain physical illnesses, can thus be interpreted in the context of the tension that exists between the disadvantages of the experience of pain and the disadvantages of the numbness which the body can facilitate by drawing on its own resources or by using external means such as drugs and medications. Hanne Seemann notes the following with reference to physically experienced pain:

> Pain is a matter between the mind and its body, and is therefore always psychosomatic, which is why the "pain" referred to here is rightly not regarded as a mental illness … The individual affected by the pain experiences and located the pain in the body, which sends out a distress signal or, in the case of chronic pain, recurring or constant messages to the mind that the latter cannot ignore because they hurt and are pressing in nature … Patrick Wall, a pioneering expert in the field of modern pain research, calls pain a "barking watchdog of health", and adds: "Pain comes when it is needed, and stays away if it is unsuitable." This alone suggests that there must be a functional system able to decide when a pain should enter the individual's conscious and when it should not.[56]

This does not mean that the body's decision is always a necessary or optimal one. Very often, however, the body can be prompted to reduce or eliminate pain through verbal instructions or vivid images conjured up in the imagination.[57]

Acquiring the ability to feel physically and also emotionally well regulated in all respects, or in other words without experiencing this process as overload, is of central importance for effective therapy.[58]

In principle, dissociative phenomena, for example resulting from a trauma (or in hypnosis) have a numbing effect on emotional and physical pain. This includes:

- amnesia,
- anaesthesia,
- age regression and progression,
- catalepsy and ideomotor movements,
- spatial distortion (*seeing things as smaller or larger than they really are*),
- time distortion (*decelerated or accelerated experience of time*),
- negative hallucination (*blanking physical reality out during daydreams*),
- reduction in experienced volume (*reducing the auditory threshold, ignoring noise*).

Traumatic experiences are often associated with wide-ranging physical reactions that present many disadvantages, particularly if they are experienced over a long period of time.

If we regard paralysis as a characteristic feature of trauma, depression (for example) can be regarded as a chronic variant of such paralysis.

The good intention of depression

"Depression is not really a state of emotional pain, but instead a state of unbearable numbness," I sometimes say to clients and their relatives. "Life feels pointless, and most of the time you're not even capable of having a good cry about it. If there were to be a 'good intention' of depression, some function or other that explains why it exists – it might be to numb some overpowering pain that was there before-hand. This is generally linked to loneliness and feeling completely alone. There's often a clear starting point in childhood; a newborn spends time in an incubator, a child experiences humiliation or grief alone or was not wanted in the first place. Depression is what numbs the pain. When the depression eases up, the ability to feel returns, and often also part of the pain from before: sadness, despondency or anger. But now it's different to before; there are people there to accompany you. I believe that you can afford to allow yourself to feel. Ask your brain to ensure that while progress is being made, you never feel too much and nothing ever gets out of hand, so that you never again become paralysed."

The good intention of mania

A politician told me that he had experienced a period of severe mania – the only one in his life so far – for several months after the death of his son. He was lucky firstly because he had friends who confronted him, and secondly because he – unlike most others in his situation – was capable of understanding the legitimacy of their warn-ings. He withdrew from his public offices before he could cause any significant harm to himself or others, and took himself to therapy. Based on what the man told me, I came to believe that mania also performs the function of numbing an overwhelming pain. Since then this assumption has repeatedly proven to be true.

"I'm impressed by the fact that you're doing so well, and that you're so full of strength and energy," I said to a man experiencing a phase of acute mania. "That's not something you can take for granted! I'm sure you've gone through a lot as well." "You're not wrong there!" "Can you give me any examples?" I asked. The client talked about the events that had caused him stress, and became serious. "That's caused you enormous suffering. But you wouldn't know it to look at you." "I try to hide it," he said, and looked extremely sad. "If we were to imagine some-one who was sad despite this strength and cheerfulness – can we do that?" The man answered in the affirmative and burst into tears. "If we were to imagine that the person who is so terribly sad could step out of you and place himself over there so that you can look at him, is that OK?" The man nodded and became calmer. "If we were to imagine that the person who is sometimes so wired could also go over there, on the other side, and you could see him there, is that also OK?" The man agreed and started to talk about his life in a calm, clear, powerful voice.

Addiction too can be interpreted as the numbing of a pain that was previ-ously there and would probably also still be there if the addictive behaviour were discontinued.

The good intention of addiction

Parents regularly bring their children and teenagers to therapy and explain to me that they are addicted to computers, gaming, their mobile phone, or something similar. Attempts by the therapist to encourage the young people to reduce their screen consumption often prove difficult. The therapist can alternatively tell the parents and their children that screen consumption performs an important function, because it typically numbs an underlying pain that probably relates to hurt, loss, and loneliness. He can ask how long the criticised behaviour has been going on, and when it stepped up in intensity and led to conflicts within the family. The subsequent discussions regularly uncover details of break-ups, bereavements, and other pivotal experiences of loss or humiliation. This firstly stops arguments over the question of "how much" screen consumption is permitted. The therapist can then start to work on the stressful events. Screen consumption typically then reduces without this issue even playing a major part any more.

The good intention of bipolar disorder

The term "bipolar disorder" appears to suggest that an affected individual can only be manic or depressive, or at most somewhere between the two. Medications are used to try and keep the individual at the midpoint of the two poles. This reduces the "bipolar patient" to a single dimension (Figure 3.6).

Instead of talking about bipolar disorder, one could also talk about tripolar disorder,[59] where the third pole is traumatically induced fear or another emotional stress. It dominates whenever mania or depression have receded from the foreground. This means that everything starts with pain – pain that is so overwhelming that the body numbs it in order to ensure that the individual is capable of action. This can be achieved in different ways.

A body can produce mania, which is a highly active and often euphoric state, potentially linked with delusional hubris. In this case the pain is numbed by an enormously positive experience and any number of distractions. The advantage is that this state is extremely pleasant, but the disadvantage is that it consumes so much energy that it cannot be maintained in the long run.

If the mania can no longer be maintained, the body can achieve numbness by means of depression, which is a state with very little in the way of emotions, bodily sensations, drive or mental capacity. The advantage is that this state can be maintained even with very low reserves of energy, but the disadvantage is that it is extremely unpleasant and the person is barely capable of action, with the reduction in activity leading to self-harming acts and in particular omissions.

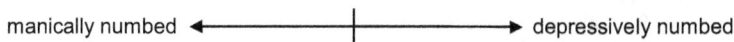

manically numbed ◄————————————┼————————————► depressively numbed

Figure 3.6 Bipolar disorder – switching between opposite forms of numbing traumatic pain

fear, pain, traumatic memory

"adjusted",
numbed by
using medications

manically numbed ⟷ depressively numbed

goal of therapy:
capable of feeling, sensitive to pain and beauty,
but protected against overload

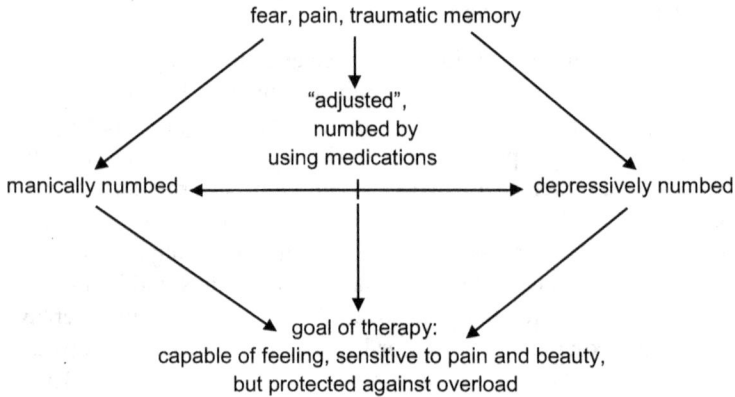

Figure 3.7 Bipolar disorder: Numbing or transforming traumatic pain

Another option available is the use of addictive substances to numb the pain. Many individuals diagnosed with bipolar disorder misuse alcohol, sleeping pills, and sedatives, which can be interpreted as an attempt to self-medicate. The disadvantage is the potential for the body to suffer harm and for the individual's social life to be adversely affected, and the potential advantage is the temporary regulation of manic or depressive tendencies, as well as the reduction in the underlying pain.

A similar effect is achieved in clinical settings using medications. The advantage here is that counselling is provided and the dosing of the substances in question is somewhat under control. The disadvantage is that although many clients suffer less anxiety, they also lose the capacity to feel joy and to feel alive thanks to the breadth of their emotional experiences.

The good intentions of mania, depression, and addiction can be acknowledged, but the implementation strategies are not particularly helpful. The aim of therapy is to regulate the suffering in such a way that it never becomes overwhelming, and the numbing strategies that have previously been dominant thus become unnecessary.

This results in the scheme shown in Figure 3.7.

The good intention of psychosis

In a crude approximation, an individual's psychotic experience can be regarded as similar to a vivid night-time dream. Yet it differs from such a dream in that it takes place during the daytime, lasts for longer, and involves a certain amount of interaction with others. Other people and current events are integrated into the story told by the dream. Many clients who experience psychotic episodes talk about childhood experiences of neglect, violence, and humiliation. Psychotic episodes can be interpreted in the following way.

Some individuals who as children were exposed to enormous interpersonal stresses within their families (or in other words without being able to escape the problem) use their talent for dreaming in order to run away from the pain of violence and loneliness into a world of dreams, even at a young age. It's like when an unhappy and lonely person switches on the television to distract himself from his sorrow. Since an individual in this situation has regular occasion to feel pain, he learns to live in a dream world almost continuously for long periods of time. If the dream world is more attractive than the physically experienced world because it numbs his spiritual pain, his internal self will prefer it to reality. Sometimes positive dreams turn into nightmares that can be exceptionally unpleasant; as we know from the nightmares we have at night, however, the situation that is experienced appears to be so real that the dreamer cannot find a way to escape and return to other people's reality (which is perhaps more bearable). If something reminds this individual of the original stress at a later date (or in other words the traumatic experience of the initial situation is "triggered"), it may be the case that a permanent dream state is involuntarily switched on as a conditioned response and a defence against the current and earlier remembered pain.

Lots of people can choose between a number of different options for numbing pain. In the case of patterns described as manic-depressive, subjectively speaking a manic phase is significantly more pleasant than a depressive phase. Yet the manic numbing strategy consumes an enormous amount of energy, whereas depression is possible also and in particular in exhausted states. This is why people crash out of a manic phase into a depressive phase, but hardly ever the other way round. Lots of people living in manic, depressive, or manic-depressive states use addictive substances as an additional pain-numbing strategy.

People whose spectrum of pain-relief strategies includes psychotic episodes also often use addictive substances. As far as I can see, "drug-induced psychosis" tends to occur not when the addictive substance is being taken continuously, but when it is removed, or in other words when the previous pain-relief strategy no longer works and must be replaced with another. If antipsychotics or other psychotropic drugs that suppress the emotional experience are then prescribed, a permanent dream state sometimes becomes unnecessary as a numbing agent, and the body decides to accept the medications as a means of regulating the pain instead of the psychotic dreams or the psychoactive substances that were previously consumed.

If this model is deployed, the question that arises is how trauma therapy can replace physical and emotional numbing with more helpful types of pain regulation.

The way back from paralysis and numbness towards feeling and acting may be associated with fears, grief, the return of suppressed memories, physical pains, or other symptoms. Part of therapy involves encouraging people – if necessary – to embark on this route, and another part of therapy, which must at the same time be borne in mind, involves ensuring that the initial stress that may result from resolving the paralysis and numbness remains as minimal as possible and never gets out of hand. The latter can be achieved *inter alia* using suggestive methods, or in other words by generating positive expectations and a helpful interpretation of any symptoms that emerge. The following parable can be used for clients who are dealing with depression or other consequences of trauma.

Storm at sea and the polar ocean

I'd like to tell you a story about grief, trauma, and depression. The way I imagine it is that a long time ago, you and the ship of your life were caught in a storm at sea that was so violent that you thought, "I'll never make it through! I'll go down with the ship!" Since you thought that there was no longer anything left to rescue, you went below deck to await your end. There you saw a red button with the words: "Do not press! Danger!" Because nothing mattered any more anyway, you pressed it and boom! The raging sea around you was transformed into a polar wasteland. Your ship was caught in the pack ice!

You were probably thinking, "I'm safe!" Now you would no longer sink to the bottom of the sea! But you quickly realised that it was bitterly cold and lonely, there was nothing to eat, and there was no possibility of getting anywhere.

Eventually the storm passed, the sun was shining on the ice and the ice started to crack. The ship rocked itself free and sailed through the fragmenting ice floes, out to sea! You were probably thinking, "I'm safe!" Then you noticed how the ship was rocking on the waves, and how water would sometimes spray over the railing into your face. And although the waves weren't particularly big, and although you knew that they were simply part of sailing at sea, the rocking now reminded you of the big storm. "For God's sake! Please let there not be another storm like the one back then! What about if a wave knocks me overboard? I'll steer the ship back into the ice, that way at least I won't go down with the ship!"

Once you'd arrived in the ice, you noticed again how cold and hopeless it was, so you steered the ship back out to sea again, got scared again, sailed back again, sailed out again, backwards and forwards...

Pass on the following greeting to your mind. You are not really in the middle of an ocean full of waves; instead, the ocean full of waves is inside you, and your mind can steer the waves so that they never get too big, so that nothing ever gets out of hand, so that you always remain on board, and so that you stay on course and make progress. Ask your mind if it can do that for you. In your opinion, what does your mind think about that idea?[60]

A desire for harmony as an attitude of protecting others and oneself in order to avoid pain can result in distressing confusion in romantic and parent–child relationships or at the workplace. The metaphor "Lumbago" can be used to present the option of daring to embark on a path away from a well-meant but unhelpful "compensatory posture" of this kind.

Lumbago

It was like there was a jinx on me. I had this terrible pain. I thought, "It's best if I just don't move any more. The only way I can bear it at all is if I hold my arm out a bit, pull my right shoulder up a little, allow the left shoulder to hang down and at the same time lean forwards ever so slightly." If I was careful, I could even walk over to the telephone or the door. But how was I supposed to pick up the telephone or press down the door handle without changing my posture? Every wrong movement caused me terrible pain. On the other hand, what did "wrong movement" even mean? The longer I remained in my unnatural protective posture, the worse the tension in my muscles and the worse the pain afterwards. And so if my salvation was to some extent a trap – what did that mean? I decided to carry out an experiment. Instead of searching for a position in which my body felt good, I assumed the most painful posture that I could bear over an extended period, and stayed there. To my surprise, the pain subsided after just a few minutes. My range of movement had increased. Then I leaned into the pain once again – the worst pain I could manage to bear. It subsided again after a while, and I could move myself more freely. I repeated the procedure probably six or eight times. Then it was as though the lumbago had been conjured away![61]

Feet against the radiator

Your mind knows what it's like when your feet are frozen and numb after a long winter's walk. It also knows that to begin with it will hurt for a little while when you warm your feet up against the radiator. It knows that this is a transitional stage; soon your feet will thaw out, and then they'll be warm. It's like that when the mind thaws out ...[62]

The anecdote "Barbarossa"[63] can also be used to resolve trauma-conditioned paralysis and defence reactions.

3.3.3 Conflicts, double binds, and counter double binds

A conflict exists when an individual believes that he is obliged to choose between several possible behaviours that are all associated with significant disadvantages and are therefore regarded as unacceptable (or in other words as a "problem").

Minor conflicts are along the lines of "biscuits or chocolate", whereas serious conflicts are along the lines of "plague or cholera". All possible behaviours are assessed as negative by the person experiencing the conflict. Yet "assessing" involves measuring something against certain values, which are based on the community of values to which the person belongs. A conflict is therefore when every behaviour that the client might choose in relation to a person or group that is important to him would involve him feeling unrecognisable to himself. From an internal perspective he would thus be acting contrary to his identity or integrity, and from an external perspective he would be calling into question his role in relation to the important person or group. Whether the person or group actually judges him is of secondary importance as far as the experience of conflict is concerned. The crucial factor is that he is disparaged by the image of this person or group in his head.

Since we perform a separate role in every group to which we belong, we have a different experience of identity in each of them. This includes slightly different sets of values and attitudes of self-awareness as well as differing levels of remorse (i.e. a clear or guilty conscience) in relation to our behaviour vis-à-vis the people or groups involved.

If the client believes (perhaps for good cause) that her dilemma is perceived in a similar manner by several people within the system, we can talk about an external conflict. If she is of the opinion that the conflict is not plainly perceived by others, we refer to an internal conflict. Ultimately, every external conflict also has a significant internal impact, and every internal conflict has a more or less significant external impact. For example, people suffering from what are known as compulsive disorders experience significant internal conflicts, which they typically conceal from most other people. Nevertheless, their demeanour towards others, and therefore the way in which they are seen and treated by others, is often shaped by these internal conflicts.

A typical external conflict is as follows: "Should I stay with my husband or move in with my affair partner?" A typical internal conflict is as follows: "Should I stick to my diet at the party, or eat crisps and chocolate and drink alcohol – or should I not go to the party in the first place so that I stick to my diet?"

At first glance, internal conflicts have nothing to do with role expectations and belonging. Yet if we take a second look, it turns out that not going to the party is linked to an experience of having one's sense of belonging called into question, and the same is true for not eating and drinking like the other guests. Not sticking to the diet is linked to challenging the standard of beauty set by one's partner, one's mother, or the parts of society one wishes to please. Breaking the rules may mean contravening the principles by which one was raised, and therefore feeling less welcomed by the "parents in one's head". It may also mean jettisoning the principles one has imparted to one's children or other people, thereby appearing untrustworthy to oneself or to them (the physical originals or merely their images in one's head).

Anyone who construes life as a conflict believes themselves to be playing a game that they cannot win. Regardless of what they do, they are harmed by it – or (which amounts to the same thing) they harm others and betray their values. The idea of errors or guilt is of central importance in this worldview. This thus also provides for the option of construing conflicts in such a way that the other party is guilty, regardless of what they do.

In the 1960s, Watzlawick, Weakland, and Jackson came up with the notion that the emergence of schizophrenia could be traced back causally to the communication of double binds. Although this model for the emergence of schizophrenia is widely rejected nowadays, this does not alter the significance of his observation that communication which repeatedly expresses irreconcilable ideas at the same time in a paradigmatic fashion, which demands a comprehensively appropriate reaction, and which prohibits the challenging of this communication can cause enormous social harm.[64]

One example might be if a mother utters terms of endearment to her child with a spiteful voice and rough stroking motions, and then complains about the child's ungratefulness for not reciprocating her devotion and love. If the child addresses the incongruence of her behaviour, this is invoked as evidence of his ill will. In this instance, the contradictory aspects of the communication are split between the verbal and non-verbal parts of the message. These aspects may also switch over if the mother talks about the child's wickedness with a soft, sad voice.

Of course, our internal self-communication sometimes resembles a double bind of this kind. If I break my diet, I'm pathetic; if I stick to my diet at the party, I'm a bore; if I don't go to the party, I'm an outsider. If I find fault with myself for being negative because I think that all of the options are bad, this proves how extraordinarily negative I really am.

Milton Erickson also uses the term double bind, but from a somewhat different angle. He typically refers to therapeutic double binds,[65] or in other words a type of intervention where both sides of an ambivalence are given new associations (with either a positive or a negative value). From the client's perspective, the dilemma that has been engineered to date is challenged in a complex fashion, and she is called upon to reassess in every respect her situation, which to date has been regarded as a conflict. The complexity of the suggestions makes it necessary for the client to carry out this reassessment intuitively rather than cognitively. This often means that she adopts a helpful new attitude.

Small spiders, big spiders

A client once said to me, "I'm not very good at standing up for myself. I'm probably too weak." She had often talked about the fact that she was short, that her voice was quiet, and that she was often overlooked and ignored. "Maybe," I responded. "Last week I cleaned my seminar room. There was a big fat spider in the corner. I blew on it to see whether it was still alive, but it didn't move an inch. When I picked it up, I noticed that a very small cellar spider with spindly legs had been hiding behind it, and was still very much alive. These teeny tiny cellar spiders can gobble up large spiders, even the big fat hairy ones that so many people are scared of. They spin a sticky web around them until they're not moving any more. Then they pounce on them. Zebra spiders are even smaller than cellar spiders. They stay still in one place. When a large spider approaches them, they jump straight upwards and land right on their victim's back. Then they have all the time in the world to get stuck into them." The woman smiled and said nothing. The issue of "being small" was now forgotten.[66]

The fact that the woman is physically weaker than those with whom she is in conflict is acknowledged. Her short stature is emphasised, and not dressed up with concepts such as "daintiness" or "cuteness". The conflict is not trivialised, but instead dramatised. Yet a distinction is also made: small and quiet does not mean defenceless or harmless. The intervention can also be used within the framework of therapy for arachnophobia (fear of spiders).

My friend, the sound

A man who was an experienced tai chi practitioner once developed tinnitus. He explained that he overcame the problem by accepting it. Over a period of several days, he used it repeatedly as a focus to enter a meditative trance, during which he imagined that the sound was his friend. Then the sound disappeared.

I told his mother about it. She said that she had also suffered from tinnitus.

"I said to my ear, 'Feel free to give the odd chirp, but leave me in peace!'" The sound had then disappeared.

A therapeutic double bind is used as a suggestion to resolve the ambivalence that expresses itself in the symptom.[67]

3.3.4 A decision – or not?

Sometimes clients ask the therapist to help them out of a particularly unfortunate situation. They explain that they are carrying on an affair with a lover behind their spouse's back, that they (and often also the two other people involved) are enormously distressed by this love triangle, but that they cannot seem to manage either to break up with one of the partners, to accept the situation as it is, or to bring about an acceptable situation in some other way. "I can't relieve you of the responsibility for taking the decision about whom you should choose," I've often said. Frequently, what the client says in response is: "No, I don't want you to – but if you could help me to make a decision – *any* decision – that would be wonderful."

The therapist can then try to do as the client asks for a while, but will eventually make the following discovery:

- If he behaves neutrally, nothing much shifts in the client's mindset.
- If he comes down on the side of one of the partners, the client internally first takes the side of that partner and then the other, or vice versa.
- If he speaks out in favour of keeping both partners, the client says it would be impossible.
- And if he discusses the option of leaving both, the client says the same.

What is to be done? If it is apparent that someone cannot decide between two partners and yet ardently desires change, I sometimes suggest to them that the time is not yet right for the decision. Therapy can nevertheless go some way towards relieving the burden on the individual in question until the point in time when he (or his partner) takes a final decision.

Picking blackberries

I often helped my parents in the garden when I was a child. I remember my father teaching me how to harvest blackberries: "Take the blackberry in your hand and gently tug on it. Not too hard, just a little tug. If it's ripe, it'll fall into your hand all on its own. Let go if it doesn't fall off by itself. It'll still taste sour."[68]

Tilling the field

During the period of time until the situation permits a decision, I propose that we should work on all the influences from your previous life, from your childhood and from previous generations of your family which might be preventing you from taking a decision or exacerbating the pain of any farewell that might be necessary. Think of it like a farmer tilling his field, or in other words ploughing and harrowing the land so that the desired crop thrives on it at a later date.

This procedure has repeatedly been found to relieve the burden on clients and to generate energy and hope, even if it does not immediately bring about change.

Getting both partners out – and the guilty conscience too!

The method of therapeutic modelling can initially be used to remove both partners from the client's head. The person who does not want to disappoint anyone, the person who is afraid of being alone, and all of the persons who are ashamed or guilty or would be ashamed or guilty of acting in line with one of the available options can subsequently be assigned to places in the room.

Once again, this procedure might not mean that the problem is necessarily solved yet, but the client will probably feel relieved on the one hand, and relatively strong and capable of action on the other.

Notes

1 Schmidt 2005, 51 *et seq.*
2 See Watzlawick's idea that, "we feel real to the extent that a significant other confirms or ratifies our self-image", Watzlawick et al. 2011, 71.
3 Schmidt 2005, 39.
4 Meyer-Erben & Zander-Schreindorfer 2021, 17.
5 Bartl 2016, reproduced from www.hager-katharina.at/grundlagen.
6 Harari 2011, 26, Dunbar 1997.
7 Schmidt 2005, 52 *et seq.*
8 See ego state therapy.
9 Summarised in Mücke 1996, 94 *et seqq.*
10 www.stanford-prison-experiment.de.
11 Molcho 1994, 189 *et seqq.*; see Eibl-Eibesfeldt 1997, 489. I use observations of this kind during therapeutic discussion in order to take the sting out of arguments about housework and to invite clients to view them with humour.
12 For further details of aphorisms as a type of intervention, see Hammel 2019a, 263 *et seq.*
13 Based on www.stefanhammel.de/blog/2008/01/16/38.
14 Astrid Vlamynck reflects on this issue as follows. "In principle, forgiving others is a good idea. But forgiveness can't be forced. Forgiveness comes automatically as a culmination when sufficient time and space has been given to all the relevant issues. Then we can know that it was unfortunately impossible for the others to do things any differently … There are very few people who genuinely want to do harm. Yet they do exist. More's the pity!" Vlamynck 2019, 136.
15 I am indebted to Alexandra Spitzbarth for this conceptual and graphical concept. Seminar discussion 2018.
16 This is illustrated by the following custom historically practised by an indigenous tribe in Alaska: in times of famine, the tribe placed members who did not contribute anything to its survival out in the wilderness. See Wallis 1994.
17 I am grateful to Sabine Müller-Löw from Mainz for this intervention.
18 See Hammel 2019a, 109 *et seq.*
19 See Beaulieu 2006, 27 *et seq.*

20 I am grateful to Ortwin Meiss for this intervention. Seminar discussion 2018; Meiss 2016, 139 *et seqq.*
21 I am grateful to Louise Beisel from Heidelberg for this intervention.
22 See the interventions "The heavenly university of love and wisdom" and "The heavenly soul cleansing" in Chapter 2, section "Inside and outside".
23 See the intervention "Packages of love" in Chapter 2, section on systemic therapy under the heading "What remains the same and what changes…".
24 See "I'll take both" in this chapter and section under the heading "New allegiances".
25 See Hammel 2016a, 53.
26 Kachler 2010, 186 *et seqq.*; Kachler 2018, 186 *et seqq.*; Kachler 2021a, 199 *et seqq.*
27 Hammel 2016a, 116.
28 See the metaphor "Clearing out the cupboard" in Hammel 2012c, 102.
29 Chapter 2, section on psychodrama, etc., "'I' as many".
30 Ibid.
31 An explanation of how plausibility can be created is provided in Chapter 2, section on hypnotherapy, "Factors affecting therapy" (Factor 2).
32 For example, the child who has not yet been conceived in the context of therapy for unwanted childlessness, in Chapter 8, section "Therapeutic modelling" (heading: "Subtraction, addition, and transformation…").
33 See "Perpetrators and victims" in this chapter.
34 See Hammel 2020, 32.
35 See section on psychodrama, etc., "Inside and outside".
36 The Old Testament idea of loving your enemy is not an expression of infectious friendliness. Instead, it is a clever transformation of the desire for revenge, perhaps to prevent retaliatory violence and feuds: "If your enemy is hungry, give him food to eat; if he is thirsty, give him water to drink. In doing this, you will heap burning coals on his head, and the LORD will reward you." See Proverbs 25, 21–22, NIV. By quoting this, Jesus establishes the principle of "loving your enemy" at the same time as suspending the moral dualism in the impartiality of God: "But I tell you, love your enemies and pray for those who persecute you, that you may be children of your Father in heaven. He causes his sun to rise on the evil and the good, and sends rain on the righteous and the unrighteous." Matthew 5, 44–45, ibid.
37 Andrew Solomon in www.esquire.com/news-politics/news/a27628/ notes-on-an-exorcism. For further details of spatially and energetically oriented perspectives on depression in Shamanism, Buddhism, Christianity, and Western philosophy, see Alz 2022, 173 *et seqq.*
38 The spread of conspiracy theories and the radicalisation of some of their proponents during the COVID19 crisis is evidently attributable to the need to be able to pinpoint and tackle hazards in an ambiguous situation. Like the conditioning of trigger reactions in overburdening situations, the development of individual and collective delusional systems also appears to me to serve the purpose of rendering intangible threats manageable.
39 youtu.be/rdl3inJYbQk, Min. 20:20 *et seqq.*; 22.10.2020, see Hammel et al. 2021, 11.
40 Hammel et al. 2021, 12 f., see previous footnote. Cyrulnik refers to an experiment evaluated by his colleagues Patrick Clairvoy and Michel Delage from the University of Toulon for the French army. Delage worked as a professor in the French army's ambulance service and as the head physician at the Saint-Anne Military Hospital in Toulon. I was unable to verify whether the experiment did in fact take place as stated.
41 See Hammel 2014a, 151.
42 Hypnosystemic interventions for couples suffering from the consequences of trauma can be found in Hammel 2019a, 152 *et seqq.*, Hammel 2020, 83 *et seqq.*; Hammel et al. 2015, 111 *et seqq.*; Hammel et al. 2021, 132 e.*t seq.*, 135, 137 *et seq.*; Hammel et al. 2020, 66; Hammel 2019, 208 *et seqq.*
43 See Chapter 8.
44 Hammel 2016a, 27.

45 See Chapter 2, section on hypnotherapy, "The cycle of memory and expectation".
46 Nina Hagen, TV-Glotzer, www.songtexte.com/songtext/nina-hagen/tv-glotzer-3bd80434. html.
47 Schmidt 2004, 184 *et seq.*
48 Seemann 2022, 109 *et seq.* Claudia Weinspach says that, "Paradoxically enough, acceptance can be used as a compelling force for change." Short & Weinspach 2007, 242.
49 Schmidt 2005, 11.
50 Schmidt 2005, 85 *et seq.* Martina Groß and Vera Popper put it the following way: "We need a 'not only but also' approach when dealing with our ambivalences." They recommend simultaneously valuing different and apparently contradictory options for interpreting the situation and acting. See Groß & Popper 2020, 85. Mechthild Reinhard believes that people face the task of seeking a constant balance between the "reference system of the world" and the "reference system of paradise". The former stands for the viewpoint that there is an objective world, and the latter for the framework of the world's subjective perception and attribution of meaning. Conflicts of loyalty between apparently immutable realities and external requirements as well as own needs are often related to this phenomenon. It is helpful to view oneself from a sufficient distance, from the perspective of a well-meaning observer, in order to honour equally the various sides of the experience. See Reinhard 2018; www.hager-katharina.at/grundlagen.
51 See Chapter 2, section on hypnotherapy, "Pacing and leading".
52 Ibid., "Factors affecting therapy", Factor 3.
53 See Chapter 9, "Dispelling doubts and building optimism".
54 See Chapter 8, "Therapeutic spaces".
55 See sections on "Role and identity" and "Abandonment and trauma" in this chapter.
56 Seemann 2022, 26, quoting: Wall 1982.
57 Illustrative case studies can be found in Hammel 2019a, 52 *et seqq.*; Hammel 2011, 53 *et seqq.*; Fruth 2021, 235 *et seqq.*
58 See Factor 6 in Chapter 2, section on hypnotherapy, "Factors affecting therapy".
59 See Hammel 2014a, 277 *et seq.*; Hammel 2016a, 74.
60 For further details of the "storm at sea" metaphor, see Hammel 2016a, 67. For further details of the transformation of landscapes and the swapping of experienced external world and internal world, see Chapter 8, section "Therapeutic maps and landscapes"/"Idiomatic landscapes". For further details of therapeutic greetings, see Chapter 8, "Therapeutic Greetings".
61 See Hammel 2012c, 48.
62 Based on Hammel 2020, 43 *et seq.* The thawing process is sometimes accompanied not only by painful feelings, but also by unpleasant memories. For further details, see the metaphor "Ötzi from the glacier" in Hammel et al. 2021, 51.
63 Chapter 8, section "Therapeutic stories"/"Role models".
64 Weakland 1960; Watzlawick et al. 1967, 214 et seqq., 223, 239 *et seqq.*
65 Erickson & Rossi 1979, 42 *et seqq.*
66 See Hammel 2019a, 112 et seq. For additional examples of therapeutic double binds, see ibid., 118 *et seq.* 139 *et seqq.* 158 *et seq.* 188, 189, 225, 229. The story is also an example of metaphorical reframing.
67 See also the remarks on the moon ritual in "What I stroke" in Chapter 8, "Healing rituals".
68 Hammel 2012c, 60.

Part 3

Course of therapy

Following a brief exchange of greetings, a traditional systemic session rapidly moves on to clarifying the client's objectives and remit. The search for helpful ideas and appropriate solutions then commences. Paul Watzlawick differentiates the stages of work somewhat more precisely, and distinguishes between four phases of the process for developing solutions with clients:

1. defining the problem in clear and concrete terms,
2. investigating the solutions attempted to date,
3. defining clearly the objective of treatment (the solution),
4. specifying and implementing a plan for bringing about this solution.[1]

This corresponds to the following sequence of steps:

1. identifying the problem and taking a history of it,
2. taking a resource-based history and acknowledging the client's suffering and attempted solutions,
3. clarifying objectives,
4. therapeutic interventions.

The above can be used as a possible basis for structuring a therapy session. Yet sticking strictly to this order would entail a disadvantage that is more significant than might appear at first: the actual therapy is delayed. Why is that a bad idea?

What we expect routinely becomes what we experience. The start of a course of therapy generates expectations about its progress, and does so in a highly effective manner. The earlier and more purposefully the therapeutic work starts, the faster and more effective the entire process. If we want to work as effectively as possible, this means that:

- the preliminary meeting is therapy,
- the greeting is therapy,
- the clarification of objectives is therapy,
- the history-taking is therapy,
- the therapy is therapy ...

DOI: 10.4324/9781003425014-6

The following subsections do not therefore represent separate segments of the therapy session that should be clearly demarcated from each other, but different areas of focus that tend to follow on from each other, but can also be swapped around as desired. Therapeutic interventions that are primarily associated with the relevant aspect of work are therefore set out in each part of the book.

I remember an occasion many years ago when I was speaking to a potential client who was considering embarking on a course of therapeutic work to tackle a phobia, and I told her, "Therapy of this kind typically takes two or three sessions." In the moment I took this to be an expression of my skill as a therapist, but the following question came to me after hanging up: what if these courses of therapy always lasted two or three sessions for the precise reason that I always told the client it would last that long? A "time placebo" of sorts, with the unconscious ensuring that matters proceed quickly because it has received the instruction to ensure that they proceed quickly, quite by the by – that's just the way it is.

Viewed in this light, it would be worth telling people that the course of therapy will only last one session. That might damage the therapist's authority, however, because the client would start the course of therapy with an immediate feeling of scepticism about whether it could really take so short a time, and as soon as the work became more complex than was initially presumed the therapist would be under pressure to live up to his own prediction, which would also be detrimental to progress.

What has proven successful is telling clients that therapy, "typically progresses very quickly, often requiring fewer than five sessions and typically fewer than ten", together with a remark to the effect that every course of therapy is unique, and it should be obvious in the first or second session how much progress is being made. During the first session, the therapist might then express delight about how well work is progressing, and voice the conjecture that it will be possible to end the course of therapy, "earlier than expected".

Based on my observations, courses of therapy tend to last longer when a health insurance fund covers the cost of 20, 40, or more sessions than when a client is covering the cost herself. Potential reasons include the following: the client might want to make the most of the health insurance fund's coverage as something she is treating herself to (or something the health insurance fund is treating her to), the therapist might unconsciously be less ambitious in his efforts to ensure that therapy progresses rapidly, or the confirmation of 20 hours of coverage might contain a suggestion, namely that the health insurance fund does not expect progress to be any faster. Confirmations of long-term coverage would then function as a "time nocebo"; the work will last a long time because it has been implicitly announced that it will do so.

The cycle of memories and expectations has been discussed earlier on:[2]

- what we remember routinely becomes what we expect,
- what we expect routinely becomes what we experience,
- what we experience routinely becomes what we remember,

- and what we have routinely remembered, expected, experienced, and then remembered again is what we call lived experience, and what we rely on as an eternal law of the universe.

The fourth rule of effective therapy applies reliably:[3] the more that is achieved during the first session from the client's perspective, the faster the progress of the remainder of the course of therapy as a whole. This realisation, however, leads to the conclusion that a therapist, particularly during the first session, should prioritise any type of action that provides the client with an experience of having achieved a lot. The question is therefore as follows: how can we achieve the best possible therapeutic outcome in the shortest possible time?

Probably not by spending the whole of the first session on history-taking questions or questionnaires, unless these simultaneously function as effective therapy. And probably also not by providing the client with the opportunity to spend the majority of the time explaining her problem.

Instead, the time spent taking the client's history can be reduced to the bare minimum, or the history-taking process itself can become therapy.

The former results in a rapid transition from history-taking to therapy, because therapeutic interventions are interspersed in large numbers and at an early stage, wherever permitted by the progress of the history-taking process; the latter results in a merging of history-taking and therapy, using interventions that combine both in a single procedure.

Notes

1 Watzlawick refers to the fact that this order is also expressed in the Four Noble Truths of Buddhism: "of suffering, of the origin of suffering, of the cessation of suffering, and of the path leading to the cessation of suffering", Watzlawick et al. 2011, 109.
2 See Chapter 2, section on hypnotherapy, "The cycle of memory and expectation".
3 Ibid., "Factors affecting therapy".

Chapter 4

Preliminary meeting

It is logical that the preliminary meeting held by telephone and the phase during which objectives are clarified should be interspersed with therapeutic interventions. If the best possible outcomes in the first session have a positive impact on the further course of therapy, what can be better than good outcomes *before* the first session?

Manfred Prior has proposed that improvements in well-being even before the first therapy session should be announced during the preliminary meeting held by phone, and combined with a request to monitor these improvements, together with the following explanation:

> Research has now revealed that in over 70% of cases, improvements of some kind are observed between the first telephone call during which an appointment is made for counselling or therapy and the first actual session ... If you notice the same, if you find that anything at all has improved, I'd be grateful if you'd let me know, because it's something I'm very interested in, and I'll also follow up on this point when we first meet.[1]

These observations by Prior are backed up by solid evidence[2] and they also correspond to the experiences gained by many doctors, counsellors, and therapists – but it goes without saying that by making these statements, Prior does not wish simply to inform his clients, but also to encourage them to strengthen any improvements by focusing on them. According to Prior, 95% of his clients report improvements during the initial meeting.[3] He thus makes it clear that the degree of improvement can be increased if the good that is expected is announced to clients, if they are told to monitor it, and if they are told that they will be asked about it during the first meeting.

Monitor how things improve

Sometimes when talking to clients by phone I tell them about Prior's observations, explain that I strongly agree with them, point out that Prior found that the degree of improvement rose yet again when clients were asked to monitor these effects, and

DOI: 10.4324/9781003425014-7

ask them something along the lines of the following: "Please monitor whether the symptoms become less frequent, shorter or weaker, whether some of them disappear or whether two, three or all four aspects improve."

Notes

1 Prior 2006, 27, see 82 *et seqq.*
2 Ibid., 89.
3 Ibid., 30.

Chapter 5

Greeting

From a therapeutic perspective, it is of crucial importance that the client should feel that she is welcome and that the therapist (if this is indeed the case) is happy to see her right from the moment of greeting. This can be expressed through the therapist's voice, facial expressions, gestures, and words. An attractive room layout, a bunch of flowers, a glass of water or a cup of coffee can also express that the client is a welcome guest.

There are many good ways of greeting clients, and the choice undoubtedly also depends on the nature of the contact established between the therapist and client:

"Welcome!"
"It's great to see you!"
"Come on in!"

In terms of greetings, this may well be all that is needed for a positive encounter. Put another way, the greeting continues in the form of a focus on the therapeutic goal.

DOI: 10.4324/9781003425014-8

Chapter 6

Clarification of objectives

When discussing the question of how a meaningful and achievable objective can be defined in the conversation between a therapist and his client, Paul Watzlawick refers to the fact that, "in order to be solved, a problem first of all has to be a problem" and that, "The translation of a vaguely stated problem into concrete terms permits the crucial separation of problems from pseudo-problems. In the case of the latter, elucidation produces not a solution, but a dissolution of the complaint", whereby it is often the case "that one will be left with a difficulty for which there exists no known cure and which must be lived with".[1]

In the case of challenges of this kind which are insoluble from the outset, Schmidt talks not about "pseudo-problems", but instead – more respectfully – about "restrictions".[2] Problems are malleable, but restrictions are immutable. Problems have solutions, but in the case of restrictions what matters is finding a positive way of dealing with what we cannot influence.

Thematic areas where the issue of dealing with restrictions comes into play include the following:

- ageing processes,
- fragility and vulnerability to suffering,
- mortality (one's own and that of other living beings),
- knowledge about what happens after death,
- certainty about the whereabouts of missing persons,
- lack of control over other people's thinking and behaviour,
- individuals' lack of control over the development of major systems,
- events that have already occurred,
- striving for moral or aesthetic perfection,
- safety within relationships and other changing systems.

"If you can't change anything about the problem, change the way you deal with it," is a systemic slogan which – strictly speaking – talks not about problems, but about restrictions. On this level, the therapist and the client search jointly to find an answer to the question of which attitude and which behaviour are most likely to be potentially experienced by the client in relation to the immutable circumstances.

DOI: 10.4324/9781003425014-9

Instead of stating something to the effect that, "she [the client] must learn to live with the difficulty," hypnosystemic therapy prefers to find out how the story that the client tells herself about the circumstances of her life can be helpfully rearranged. The very process of clarifying objectives thus prepares the ground for the potential target condition.

> In Erickson's opinion, developing descriptions of objectives and the visions associated with them in a differentiated fashion is a task of crucial significance for the success of cooperation ... This means that the description of objectives not only clarifies that the work can start, but is instead a central phase of the interventions. The process of clarifying objectives thus becomes a process of imagining the target experience.[3]

Its purpose is therefore not only to generate information, but also to serve as an integral part of the therapy itself. Clarifying objectives helps to build up positive expectations, or in other words optimism and the motivation to develop further, and also to evolve internal images which the client will involuntarily adhere to as she proceeds further; it also helps to build up trust between the therapist and the client, and to avoid misunderstandings on the part of the therapist about what the client wants and how she wants to achieve it.

In the case of a client with tinnitus, the therapist can open the conversation as follows:

"You'd like your ear to be quiet for once, am I right?"
"You can say that again ..."
"Is there anything else in your life that needs to be quiet? Or different?"

A conversation with a client diagnosed with depression might start as follows:

"When we talked on the telephone, you told me that you suffered from depression. How do you know that?"
"My GP told me. For some time now I've had no energy to do anything at all, no joy, no interest in anything – I don't even want to leave the house ..."
"Would we be able to say that our work had delivered a good outcome if you recovered your interest in life, your motivation and your drive?"
"That'd be nice, but I don't know how you'd go about it."
"I can imagine that you're feeling quite hopeless at the moment. Perhaps I have more hope for you than you do for yourself. I propose that we try managing without any hope from you. If it's OK with you, I'll lend you my hope until you have some of your own again. What do you think?"

The therapist can say the following to a couple that has come to therapy:
"Once again, welcome! I don't know exactly what has brought you here yet. I'm going to assume that you two aren't getting along with each other particularly well,

and that you'd like things to be different and happier in the future. If you don't mind, I'd like to start things a little differently to what you might be expecting, and to ask the following question: supposing that what's been tending to go wrong between you two so far were suddenly to start going really well, how would *your* attitude to your partner differ from before? Remember, I don't want to know what your partner would do differently, but what *you* would do differently if things were going really, really well. Who wants to go first?"

Surprising phrases are often incorporated right at the start of the process of formulating objectives together, and have the potential to realign clients' attention,

- from experiencing a problem to imagining a good life,
- from suffering to shaping,
- from a painful memory to a positive expectation, and
- from knowledge of how the situation is to a search for how it could also be perceived.

Slight confusion on the part of the client as a result of this approach to starting the conversation can be extremely constructive in therapeutic terms. It means that the client is invited at an early stage to find new ways of looking at her problem, even before she has begun to explain her current perspective on it. Her patterns of thinking and behaving – which have presumably contributed to her involuntarily generating the problem – are interrupted and tentatively (in response to an offer made by the therapist) replaced with others.

It can be very useful to interrupt patterns at the start of the conversation in this way; at the same time, the therapist can ensure – by observing the client's non-verbal feedback or by asking questions – that the client also feels accepted and understood in her suffering. Especially if the therapist's verbal expressions of confidence do not directly respond to the client's suffering, it is important that his body language (i.e. his internal attitude) expresses acknowledgement of the client's suffering to date as well as interest and concern. In this therapeutic double bind between empathy (pacing) and awakening (leading), the therapist can use his voice intuitively to support both sides in turn: firstly to emphasise his acknowledgement of the client's suffering, and secondly to express hope that points to a future beyond what the client has suffered to date.

Notes

1 Watzlawick et al. 2011, 109.
2 Schmidt et al. 2010, 77 *et seqq.*
3 Schmidt 2005, 102 *et seq.*

Chapter 7

History-taking

Telling things takes time. And if there is a lot to tell, it takes a *lot* of time. If the history-taking phase is to be designed in a time-efficient manner, therapy cannot start with an invitation to the client to start telling the therapist about what has brought her there. Instead, targeted questions can be used as a structuring method.

The following questions alone often allow a large part of the client's history to be taken: "How long has it been like that for you? And what else was happening back then?"

In order to gain a more accurate understanding of the effect of these questions, it is helpful to try out the following experiment with yourself or with someone close to you.

Taking one's own history

Construct a table with three columns.

In the **first column**, write down all of the chronic stresses whose start you can pinpoint to a (more or less accurate) date. They might include physical symptoms or illnesses, but also mentally associated symptoms or syndromes such as anxiety, compulsive thoughts, depression, and depersonalisation.

In the **second column**, write down the date when the symptoms started. Add in times when the symptoms got worse (intensified, spread, transferred to other areas) or when earlier symptoms returned. If you think that you have "always" experienced the symptom, write "0". This refers to the period of time from conception until your first birthday. If you make use of this option, also note down whether a parent or grandparent experienced the symptom, and for how long.

In the **third column**, note down any experiences of feeling threatened, isolated, lost, unwelcome, or at the mercy of radical changes that might potentially have played a role at this time. If the symptoms emerged gradually, try and identify any conflict that was going on during this period. If an event has parallels with a previous major stress, add a note similar to the following: "Refer back to [age]".

Take a close look at the table. Can you find any illuminating connections? Can you develop any hypotheses on this basis regarding the emergence of the

DOI: 10.4324/9781003425014-10

symptoms? If you are unsure whether any coincidences are random or regular, draw up similar tables during your sessions with clients over the next week!

7.1 History-taking using systemic questions

The traditional – but not the only – method of taking a client's history involves the therapist asking the client a large number of questions in order to get to know the story behind the concern presented to him, and in order to track down the interdependencies within the system that can be influenced in order to …

- resolve the challenge that the client is experiencing,
- transform it into something else, or
- gain a fresh perspective on it so that it no longer bothers the client, or so that it provides a benefit that outweighs the disadvantages.

The therapist asks the client or clients certain questions out loud in order to generate fresh opportunities for thinking and acting, and asks himself certain questions in his head in order to orient himself in the process. The next section illustrates how a therapist can orient himself in the internal self-monologue that goes on during therapy. This is a network of conceptual trails representing possible routes from history-taking to intervention. The questions and points for consideration that are listed serve the purpose of laying the ground for therapeutically helpful interventions. The following sections illustrate how the therapist can use systemic questions to the client to orient himself to the client's situation and at the same time intervene in a therapeutically effective way, even at this early stage.

7.1.1 Questions which the therapist asks himself

With a view to generating ideas that lead to suitable interventions, the therapist can ask himself the following questions (shown as a numbered list) and test the following hypotheses (shown as bullet points) as a basis for a provisional problem-solving model:

1. What isn't working? (What is the symptom or problem being experienced?)
2. How does the thing that is "not working" work? How long has it been doing so? (*Question about the emergence of the problem*)

   - Trauma (*"Never again!"*)
   - Conflict (*"Regardless of how it's done, you lose!"*)
   - Crisis of orientation (*"I don't know what's true (or what's not true)!"*)
   - Bullying (*"I'm treated as someone I don't believe I am!"*)
   - Double bind (*"What meets my needs is harmful to them!"*)
   - Migration (*"I don't have a home!"*)

Whenever …? (*Question about the reactivation of the problem*)

- Trigger *("Help, it's just like it was back then!")*

Always and everywhere? (*Question about the continued existence of the problem*)

- Circularity *(Interdependencies, self-fulfilling prophecies)*
- Circular reasoning *(Assumptions that are self-affirming because they cannot be refuted)*

3. What works (or what previously worked) in the thing that "doesn't work"?
   - What is its good intention of (*Value, skill*)?
   - What is the inappropriate strategy being used to implement this intention?

How can that be described as an ambivalence?

- A goal is achieved, but at too high a price.
- Something that manifestly "does not work" (symptom) is coupled with something that "works" in a covert or overt manner (value).
- How can that be described as a misunderstanding?
- Achievement of a goal is actually prevented by the strategy intended to achieve it, or the opposite is achieved.

4. What can we couple (*associate*) with what is "not working" so that it no longer works?
   - Self reflexively speaking …
     - What is not working based on the client's former assessment (paradox: *"Don't worry – the part of you that says, 'I can't do anything,' can't do anything, as she herself says, and so she can't do you any harm."*)
     - What is not working based on a reassessment (reframing: *"I don't think your son is lazy – he's simply conserving energy."*)
   - Something else that "doesn't work" *("When I had a stomach upset and could feel that I was going to be sick, I ran to the toilet, thought about the colleague who bullies me, said to him in my thoughts, 'This is for you!' and bent over the toilet bowl. It was very liberating.")*
   - Something that "works" *("If you take the feeling you have while celebrating in the mountain village following the clean-up operation[1] and think again about being at home, what is different now?")*

5. What can we differentiate, separate, decouple (*disassociate*) so that what "doesn't work" no longer works?
   - The thing in itself *(e.g. the image from the sound of the "film of memories", the memory of exam stress from the fear of the anticipated exams)*

- Various things that "don't work" from each other *(e.g. anger at a husband and concern about a son)*
- What is not working and the ego experience *("You are not 'a diabetic'– you have diabetes. Otherwise someone with high blood pressure would be a high blood pressuriser.")*
- What is not working and the now, here, or ego experience *("If the person who has suffered from this pain to date was standing over there, how would she look?")*
- The good in what is not working from the bad in what is not working *(e.g. good intention and inappropriate strategy, helpful exception and inauspicious normal situation, good starting point and bad continuation)*

6. How can we convert what is not working into what is working *(transformation)*?

- Benefit as an indicator of risk *(headache as a sign of being overburdened)*
- Benefit for a value *(tinnitus as a reference sound for perfect pitch)*
- Transformation into a film *(see the mountain village intervention)*
- Transformation of a bodily sensation *(problem circle and resource circle,[2] transforming symptoms into emotions[3])*.

7.1.2 Problem-based history-taking

Most clients come to therapy because they are suffering from something that can be described as a problem, in the hope that therapy will help them to alleviate this pain. They expect that talking about the problem is a method of reducing the stress and perhaps even overcoming the problem. They want to talk about their problem, so that's where we start.

This part of the session can move through the following questions:

- If you had a theory about what triggered the problem, what would it be?
- How long has the problem existed?
- What was special about the time when the problem started?
- Had you ever experienced a similar type of stress beforehand? What was going on then?
- When is it more or less present? When is it there and when is it not?
- At which location or with which person are things different?
- What happens before, during, after? Who does what?
- If there was an automatic mechanism with a trigger and a reaction, what would be the trigger and what would be the reaction? Does the reaction itself trigger something (e.g. its own trigger), resulting in a stable cycle?
- If there were two voices in you, both thinking or wanting something different, what would the first say and what would the second say? If both want something good (for example protection, stimulation, autonomy, or belonging), what would their respective good intentions be?
- What could you do to make the problem worse?

It goes without saying that we are not only interested in clients' problems, but in their capabilities, the chances and opportunities that life offers them, their values, their preferences, their good memories, their positive expectations, and everything else that might exert a helpful influence on their life. That's why we enquire about these things – perhaps concentrating our questions at individual points or perhaps distributing them evenly over the entire period of therapy – and that's why we also follow up with questions if clients volunteer relevant information. True to the slogan of utilisation ("Use everything!"), it is of course the case that everything can be a resource if you look at it from the right angle. Whether or not something is a resource is a question of the lens through which you view it. Yet perceiving a value or an opportunity in something is naturally easy in some cases and much more difficult in others. A number of ideas for enquiring about resources in clients' lives are set out below.

7.1.3 History-taking of problems assigned by others

Certain individuals have not come to therapy voluntarily, or at least have not decided to come of their own accord, but have allowed themselves to be dragged along. It is often children and adolescents, but occasionally also adults, who have been pressured or forced by others to come to therapy. It might be that they don't want to talk at all about their problem or what others believe to be a problem. It's therefore a better idea to talk about something else with them.

Let's take the example of a teenager who has been brought to therapy because of his poor behaviour (in the opinion of the adults involved). The following questions can be used to guide the process for taking the history of the problems perceived by others in the adolescent's alleged or actual experience and behaviour.

- Was it your idea to come here today, or did your parents drag you here?
- Who else wants you to be here? Your teachers? The youth welfare office?
- What's their problem? What do they think is your problem?
- Am I right in thinking that you find them super annoying?
- Is it OK with you if we try to find out how you could get them to be less annoying?
- When do they annoy you most? When do they tend to annoy you less?
- If you ramp up the behaviour that makes them annoy you, they'll probably also ramp up their efforts to annoy you. That's not a great outcome for you. If you avoid the behaviour that makes them annoy you, they'd stop annoying you, but you'd have missed out on something else that is important to you. That's also not a great outcome for you. Somewhere between these two extremes is the sweet spot where on the one hand they annoy you less, but on the other hand you've done as much as possible of what is important to you, without them getting too annoying. Is it OK if we try to find out how you can get to that spot?
- There's no point in me carrying out therapy with you in the way they're imagining it. You know that as well as I do. But if I say that the therapy is over and

done with, they'll cart you straight off to the next shrink. That won't get you anywhere either. Would it be OK with you if we don't work on what your parents want us to work on, but on what is most likely to be important from your point of view? Is there anything in your life that could be even better than it already is?[4]

Adults can be asked similar questions, with a slightly different wording. The same applies to resource-based history-taking, as illustrated in the following section (again using the example of therapy for children and adolescents).

7.1.4 Resource-based history-taking

In other cases, children and adolescents have come to therapy not entirely against their will, but with a certain level of discomfort because the issue in question is loaded with shame. They would rather not talk about problems, but are desperate for their suffering to be alleviated (once again, the same naturally also applies to adults, with minor alterations). It follows that our conversation with them should not start with problems, and that it should stay away from this topic as much as possible. Instead, it should start with and primarily focus on what is going well in their life and how this can be expanded to other areas.

Resource-based history-taking can be structured using the following questions.

- What is (already) good? What are you good at? What do you like to do?
- When are things better than usual? (*Exception question*)
- What is good and better than now about the objective?
- How will you know that you have achieved the objective?
- If the conditions were the best they possibly could be as seen from now, when do you think you might achieve it?
- If you imagine looking back once you've achieved the objective, what do you think the first step would have been?
- If a fairy godmother took the problem away from you while you were fast asleep, how would you know tomorrow that it had gone? Who else would know, and how? (*Miracle question*)
- What do other people who don't have the problem do differently? What can you do in order to do something similar, but in your own unique way?
- How much will it cost?
- Assuming that the process is quicker than you previously thought, when do you think you will be ready?

7.2 History-taking using physical signals

What happens if we base the questions we ask during the history-taking conversation not on what the client verbally presents as her problem, but on the sound of her voice, the flow of her speech, her breathing, and perhaps also the way in which she clears her throat or sniffs and other non-verbal but audible clues? Visible gestures can of course also be included in this list ...

The therapist would then not necessarily need to hold off with questions about the context of the problem experience until the client has recounted a long tale of suffering in great detail, listed all the relevant factors and specified the issues that are of central importance in her opinion. The therapist could instead intervene as soon as the client signals – with a croak or a sob in her voice – that she associates stresses with the words just uttered that might provide additional information about the background to her suffering.

7.2.1 Using bodily signals to navigate problem-based history-taking

The therapist could also latch on to unusual features of the conversation, for example if the client's voice stutters, hesitates, or sounds brittle.

The following dialogue might develop within the framework of the history-taking process with a client who has raised the issue of her relationship with her body and with herself as a woman.

"Can you remember when you started not much liking your body and yourself as a woman?"

(*With a slight nasal twang:*) "When I was about eleven (*sniffing*) or twelve years old."

"What else was going on back then, when you were about eleven or twelve years old?"

"We were still living in Gelsenkirchen (*with hesitations*), and ..."

"Sorry for interrupting you. I just wanted to ask, what else do you associate with this Gelsenkirchen period?"

"It was a difficult time. My father was unemployed. We didn't have much money (*stammering*)."

"How important was money back then?"

"We often had nothing to eat (*phlegmy throat clearing*). My mother would constantly have a go at my father for not working. He drank and (*pause*) hit her."

"What you just said about your father hitting your mother seems to me like it might be important. How much does it bother you now?"

"They often used to shout at each other when we were in bed. Perhaps they thought I couldn't hear them because I (*dry throat clearing*) was asleep. But I wasn't asleep. Whenever they started shouting at each other, I was always (*pause*) afraid that he would cause her real harm. I didn't feel safe at all. I only started to feel a bit safer when he left."

"The fear you felt back then – is it still present today?"

"Even now I can't get a good night's sleep if someone else is staying over. And having someone sleeping in my bed isn't really an option, at any rate not if I want to get any rest. That's not great for my love life, of course. No one I've dated has stuck around for long."

The therapist's subsequent questions are not aimed specifically at the substance of what was said. The signs of stress in the woman's non-verbal but audible utterances are the sole factor determining the direction of his questions. Visible signals can also be taken into account, such as the wiping away of tears that are unconsciously remembered, either below or next to the eye or below the nose.

This approach ensures that the conversation gets down to the central issues much more rapidly than if the therapist first asks the client to explain everything that is on her mind, or if he bases his questions primarily on the verbal content of what has been said.

It is worth noting that this way of guiding the conversation often gets "to the nub of the matter" so quickly that therapists following this procedure should ensure that they are in a position to recognise and deal with clients' trauma responses.

Therapeutic greetings present a rapid and effective opportunity for ensuring that any stresses that come to light in this connection do not become too painful and do not harm the therapeutic process.[5] Hesitations in speech are one among many phenomena that may signal an issue experienced as traumatic. The more abrupt or frequent, the longer or the less syntactically relevant the pauses, the closer the conversation is getting to the centre of the traumatic memories.

For clarification: the obvious cause of a hesitant voice is hesitant thinking. Thinking becomes hesitant because the body becomes momentarily paralysed in a manner typical of traumatic experiences. The majority of non-essential brain functions are shut down for a shorter or longer period of time during this reaction, which affects not only thinking, but also the muscles, circulation, emotions, bodily sensations, and other functions.

The reason why this happens during therapy is because the client is reminded of the time when the stressful event occurred. When we are reminded of something, our brain simulates our experience at the time, together with all the sensory inputs and all the bodily reactions.

If we were instead observing an internal search and a weighing-up of what the client believes to be true and wants to express, the pauses in her speech would seem soft and would be syntactically more appropriate.

7.2.2 Using bodily signals to navigate resource-based history taking

It is of course also possible to take the opposite approach. In order to move the client away from stressful issues and towards something that is more likely to strengthen her, the therapist can dwell on whatever is being discussed when her voice, breathing, and manner of speaking seem freer, more vibrant, and more relaxed. Returning to the client from the previous example, if she were to mention that she sometimes spent a few days or weeks with her grandmother during her time in Gelsenkirchen, it might be the case that she exhibits more relaxed facial expressions, a larger range of motion, a more upwards gaze, and (most importantly) a more powerful, melodious, and soft voice, greater fluency of speech, and calmer breathing. The therapist could now ask the following.

"It seems to me that your grandmother is a very precious person in your life. Is that true?"
"Which memories do you associate with your grandmother?"
"Can you tell me something that was unique about your grandmother?"

Every word that the client utters while at the same time seeming more animated and mobile, speaking more calmly and breathing more freely should now be taken as a prompt to drill down with further questions. The resource experience can also be consolidated if the word during which the client looks and sounds most relaxed or happiest when answering each question is taken as a prompt for further questions:

(*Keyword: "to the zoo"*) "What was it like when your grandmother took you to the zoo?"
(*Keyword: "looked forward to it"*) "Was there anything you particularly looked forward to during these visits?"
(*Keyword: "feeding the baby goats"*) "What do you associate with the memory of feeding the baby goats?"

7.2.3 Linking the physiology of solutions with memories of problems

The therapist can now also constructively link with each other the resource and problem situations that have been identified.

"Memories are like internal films. We can ask your internal director to adapt the film of the bad things that happened in such a way as to make it better. Tell your brain that it should make this good feeling a priority for you, and perhaps make it even better. If it's OK with you, try imagining that you are taking a copy of your grandmother and the goats along with the whole feeling of being at the zoo to the girl who is lying there alone in her bedroom and listening to her parents shouting. Now the grandmother's there too, and the goats, and you've given the feeling of being at the zoo to the girl so that she can have as much of it as she wants. What's changed now?"
"The girl is now a lot more peaceful. The shouting still bothers her, but it doesn't worry her as much. Now grandma's there, and now she can also stroke the goats. That gives her something else to think about."
"What's changed for you when you look at the situation like that?"
"I also feel calmer."

"Yes. You're breathing a lot more calmly. Your face looks more relaxed. You aren't looking down as much. It seems to me that you're moving more freely, and now you've also smiled a little for the first time ..."

"I do feel better when I think about it like that."

"If you imagine to yourself how the girl is now feeling so much better, and if we take another copy of the grandma, the goats and the feeling of being at the zoo into a situation where you'd brought someone home you really liked, but you didn't let him stay the night, and now the grandma is in the room next door and the goats are playing in the hallway ... how is that?"

"If grandma and the goats are there, then it's OK, he can stay."

"I can see that you're now looking a lot calmer than when you first told me about the problem before. It's a big difference. Now you're breathing more calmly, and your voice sounds a lot more vibrant. Before there was a jangling note in your voice, but now it sounds powerful and rich..."

"I really do feel better now ..."

"I'm sure that it will work not just when we're sitting here and imagining it, but also if you have a man staying over. If you put the grandma and the goats somewhere nearby, things will be different. If things hadn't changed, there wouldn't be a difference between before and now, and there really is a huge difference!"

"You're probably right ..."

The therapist tells the client to ask her brain to make the helpful internal film of the zoo visit a priority. There is a reason for the somewhat clumsy phrasing: if the addressee of the instruction is an authority in the third person (the "brain") rather than the client herself ("you"), the instruction is carried out by involuntary authorities. We can forestall the inhibiting effects that might go hand in hand with the scepticism of authorities close to waking consciousness by asking whether it might also be possible to listen to the parents arguing while experiencing the feeling of being at the zoo. The memory of the resources from the visit to the zoo is associated with the traumatic triggering situation by incorporating the grandma, the goats, and the feeling of being at the zoo into the stressful memories and asking how this changes the experience of the girl from back then and the client of today. The memories of being at the zoo are subsequently linked to the situations that are currently experienced as a challenge. Then the therapist asks what changes this brings about in the client as the person she experiences herself to be in the imagined situation. The therapist makes the plausible suggestion that the changes that have been observed will also apply in situations experienced as real. By enquiring about and describing the solution-associated bodily reactions (of the girl from back then, of the woman who has a man in her bed, and of the client in the therapy session), this procedure strengthens these reactions. The client can be asked how the girl from back then will react if she ...

- sees how things are going better for her now,
- learns how, as the client, she solved her problem with her boyfriend,

- finds out how, as the woman with the boyfriend, she reacts when she notices how the girl feels better,
- notices what changes for her, as the client in the therapy session, when she experiences how things are going better for her as the woman with a boyfriend or as the girl from back then,
- discovers that each of these people feels better when they notice that the others are feeling better.

During a second (and third and fourth) stage, circular questions can be used to explore how the different imagined people react when they each notice that the others are now feeling even better because they can see how the client or the other imagined people in the room are feeling ...

7.2.4 History-taking with ideomotor signals

The process of taking a client's history using ideomotor signals is familiar from work with hypnosis. In most cases, questions are addressed to the client's unconscious by asking him to move individual fingers to answer "yes" or "no". In the simplest possible case, one finger signal is assigned the meaning "yes", and another the meaning "no". For a more differentiated approach, five fingers can be assigned the following meanings:

- yes,
- no,
- I don't know,
- I don't want to say,
- there's no answer to that.

The last of these options may mean one of two things:

- The question is based on false assumptions.
- The question is to be answered in the affirmative from one perspective, but in the negative from another.

The process for agreeing on finger signals involves placing the client in a trance using traditional hypnosis-based methods. Then her unconscious is asked to give a signal for each of the answers listed above; these signals will henceforth retain these meanings. It is a good idea for the therapist to jot down the signals so that there is no confusion over which answer is meant. It is furthermore possible for the signals to be reused in later sessions. If the therapist is tuned into their meaning, there is no need to repeat the procedure for agreeing on them; the client's unconscious will not forget them.

The procedure for agreeing on finger signals will be quicker and clearer if the therapist asks the client first to move all of her fingers and then to keep them all still except for the finger that the unconscious has in each case chosen as the "yes" finger, "no" finger etc. This procedure has proven successful even if no trance whatsoever is induced, provided that it is integrated into an active–alert dialogue within the framework of hypnosystemic therapy. The answers provided by the client's unconscious via the fingers while the client is in a state experienced as active and alert turn out to be just as reliable as those obtained during a trance session.

It goes without saying that other bodily reactions can also be agreed upon instead of finger signals. If more than five possible answers are required, both hands or combinations of several finger movements can be used to express additional options.

For example, questions starting with "how many" could be asked. The following would then be agreed:

- no fingers means zero,
- one to ten fingers mean one to ten respectively,
- a fist means "more than ten",
- two fists mean "more than a hundred",
- fists with thumbs extended mean "approximately".

If necessary, separate prompts can be used to query hundreds, tens, and units.

The ideomotor questioning method can also be associated with the concept of the tetralemma for decisions in a situation experienced ambivalently or polyvalently. In order to do so, one finger is associated with each of the following …

• "the first"	(e.g. "yes"),
• "the second"	(e.g. "no"),
• "both"	(e.g. "on the one hand yes, and on the other hand no"),
• "neither"	(e.g. "this is about something else entirely"),
• "none of that, and not even that"	(e.g. a paradoxical resolution, a fundamentally different question, a joker)

A substantive response is obtained by asking the unconscious, "Now please tell the client's conscious mind what this is all about!"

Using ideomotor signals

A woman explained that cracks had appeared in her half-timbered house. She'd had a structural engineer, a geologist, and other specialists out to look at them, and they'd all assured her that they did not pose any risk. Nevertheless, she found the situation uncanny, and was toying with the thought of selling the house she lived in and loved. She could not explain where the uncanny feeling came from, but it was really bothering her.

"If your intuition or another authority is telling you to worry, there's undoubtedly a reason for that. Let's see what we can find out in this connection," I proposed. We agreed on finger signals so that we could ask her internal authority – the source of her disquiet – what it knew about the situation.

Her unconscious used all four of the finger signals we had agreed upon in turn, and gave the following answer.

The foundations were not the problem, and nor were the roof truss, the timber framing, or the filling between the timbers – the problem lay with the soil below the foundations. There were no voids below the foundations, but there were differences in the level of soil moisture, resulting in the movement that had caused the cracks.

I suggested to the woman that she should find a dowser or someone with scientific training to verify whether this was true. If he confirmed her hypothesis, she could consider regulating the balance of moisture in the soil below the house, perhaps by adding a drainage system, by drilling a well or by installing a water tank with the option of pumping water out or injecting water in. The woman agreed to this course of action. Regardless of what emerged, she now felt a significant sense of relief as a result of focusing on specific possibilities for interpreting the situation and taking action, and feeling able to position herself in relation to these possibilities. A few weeks later she said that the session had helped her to see the matter in a new light. She planned to stay in her home, and felt good about her decision.

7.3 History-taking using life opportunities

Instead of the term "parts of the personality", which is popular in other forms of therapy, I prefer to use the phrases "options", "life opportunities", "the people who you could be," or "the people you could experience yourself as being".

From a hypnosystemic perspective, the "people" discovered during therapy are not the outcome of an analysis of immutable circumstances (e.g. subpersonalities that appear constant), but instead a construct that may differ from session to session and may also change over the course of a session.

Let's suppose that a client reports during the phase of clarifying objectives and taking a history that she wants to conquer the habit of eating "too much, too late and also too unhealthily" every evening. We might shape the history-taking process on the basis of her verbal or non-verbal feedback.

7.3.1 History-taking on the basis of verbal feedback

Let's start by examining how the history-taking process can be designed on the basis of the therapeutic objectives that the client has expressed verbally.

1. After picking up on the (negative) objective formulated by the client, the therapist can ask her to remove from herself and assign a place in the room the person who eats "too much, too late and too unhealthily" every evening.

2. The therapist can ask the client to describe this person: "When you see her over there, how is she standing? How does she look? How do you think she's feeling? What is she lacking, or what is she searching for?" The client will experience ever more clearly how she feels without this person; either she feels better, and this result can then be stabilised, or she feels worse, and then the therapist can determine what lies behind the habit of eating in the evening and explores it in greater depth. (Let's assume the second is the case for now.)

3. The client might say, "She seems restless. She wants to take her mind off things. Being alone makes her nervous. She's lonely." The therapist can ask, "How old is she?" or, in more detail, "If you make her younger and younger, until she reaches the age she comes from, how old is she?" And in yet further detail, "What did she experience back then that makes her so lonely?"

4. The therapist can also ask,

> "The person who eats a lot is over there, and you are here. How do *you* feel?"
> "Somehow I feel terribly sad."
> "Is it OK if you put the person who feels sad next to you?"
> "Yes, she can stand there."

5. The therapist can now ask what's going on with the person who feels sad and is standing next to the client (repeating Step 3, but using a different person removed from the client) or investigate how the client is feeling now that the person who feels sad has been removed from her (repeating Step 4 in structural terms).

6. The therapist can now also introduce a person who represents approximately the positive opposite of the initial negative objective that was formulated: "Supposing that out of a world where everything is possible, the person who you are when you eat *early, moderately and healthily* in the evening arrives ..."

7. As a way of countering any potential objections, he can emphasise the very real possibility of achieving the objective: "... in *comparison* to everything you have known up until now, *really* remarkably early, *surprisingly* moderately and *genuinely* healthily, *regardless of where* she finds the ability to do it. Perhaps she is *genuinely surprised* by herself ..."

8. He can lend positive connotations to the objective that has been formulated: "... *pleasantly* surprised at the *happy* and *carefree* way in which she does it ..."

9. At the same time, he can incorporate anything that emerged during the history-taking phase in relation to the origin or context of the problem. He can focus on positive wordings of the objective, or, in keeping with the idea of pacing and leading, transition from negative to positive wordings: "I believe it's the person who – instead of being *fidgety* or *nervous* is entirely *at rest in herself*; who is beyond *relaxed*, and that's why instead of *taking her mind off things*, for example, she feels agreeably powerful *in her innermost self*; and who, although she might sometimes also feel *sad*, probably no longer needs to, who trusts in chance because instead of the *loneliness* that was previously

there, she experiences in herself (wherever she gets it from) a pleasant sense of *belonging*: feeling loved, welcome, and at home in herself.

10. The therapist can ask the client to describe the posture, facial expressions, and other characteristics of this person or (if she can't see her) to guess how she might look and to be surprised at what changes when she puts herself in her place.

If the client comes to therapy and says that she has spent all week thinking about what she'd like to say during the session, but that now she's here, she can't remember any of it, the therapist can ask the client to take the person out of her who "can't remember any of it now". This would be a consistent implementation of the strategy of history-taking on the basis of verbal feedback, as described above. If the client is not able to specify an objective for the time being, he can start by using "not remembering any of it" as a negative objective, or in other words the condition the client wishes to move away from, since another side of her had prepared for the session and also brought her here in order to enter into conversation with the therapist.

7.3.2 History-taking on the basis of non-verbal feedback

Let's move on to an examination of how to design the process of taking a client's history on the basis of bodily reactions.

1. The therapist can also observe the woman's posture, manner of speaking, and voice, and ask her:

   "Imagine you could split yourself up into several people, and imagine the person who talked in such a hesitant, quiet manner just now stepping out of you. She's standing here before you. How does she look?"
   "Er – confused?"

2. The therapist can endorse the client's response by continuing as follows:

   "Yes, she looks confused! How is she standing?"
   "Indecisively, somehow?"
   "Yes, that's a definite possibility. She is standing there indecisively! In our imagination, we can divide her into several people: a person who wants one thing, another who wants something else, another who wants several things that contradict each other, and another who doesn't have any idea what she wants. What do you think, do they look the same or different?"
   "Different."

3. The therapist can suggest, "Why don't you try describing them to me? For example, how does the person look who wants one thing …", and the client describes the person in question.

The therapist can continue to watch her body language. As soon as a distinction is made between her and the person who is confused, she might seem more with it, and while she is describing the different people in front of her, she might seem to gain more and more power and clarity.

4. He can tell her this and ask her to describe what feels different when the person who is confused has been taken out of her and differentiated into many persons. While she describes what feels different, her bodily reactions and her voice might become even more powerful and clear, and her manner of speaking more fluent. The therapist can tell her again what he's observed while she's talking about how she feels in herself. "Oh, really? Yes, that's right!" A smile might spread over the client's face for the first time. "Perhaps you even have a smile at your disposal now!" the therapist could comment in a friendly fashion, thereby reinforcing precisely this tendency.

5. The therapist can continue to pay attention to whatever is communicated non-verbally. On the one hand the client appears relieved, but on the other hand pain that might have been numbed by the confusion may also emerge once the confusion has lifted. It's possible that a sad-sounding quiver might appear in the client's voice. Perhaps she clears her throat with a phlegmy sound, sniffs, or sounds nasal or rubs her face as though wanting to wipe away a tear. The therapist could say, "Supposing that there was someone inside you who felt sad, where could we put her?" Or alternatively, "If the person who's rubbing the area below her eye, and whose voice sounds a bit different, whatever that might mean, were to put herself over there and you were to look at her, how would she look?" The client might say that the person is looking at the ground, that she seems tired, that she's sad or similar. At the same time, she herself seems more alert and in a better mood, and her gaze is more upwards. (If the therapist were to say, "You just rubbed your face, which must mean this, that and the other …" he might offend the client and receive the following answer: "I simply felt an itch," which would put an end to the conversation.)

6. The therapist can express an interest in any further improvement in her well-being and strengthen the latter, or continue the history-taking process by asking, "If we examine the sad person over there, how old does she look? What do you think she's sad about?" And the client will tell him the story behind the sadness that emerged from behind the confusion.

During this procedure, the therapist pays almost no attention to the substance of what the client is telling him, but instead concentrates predominantly or almost exclusively on how she tells it. Anything suspected of being an expression of stress is personified and dissociated from the client, and described as something outside her. Describing it makes it possible to experience it and yet perceive it as distinct from her.

If symptoms of stress emerge one after another (sadness after "not remembering any of it", anger after sadness, helplessness after anger etc.), this procedure is typically (or in other words until the client expresses the wish not to do so) repeated until the stress experienced by the client progressively lessens.

In practice, it is advisable to use a mixture of history-taking methods based on verbal and non-verbal approaches. Focusing on non-verbal alternatives typically helps the client to drill down to the key points and experience a sense of relief more rapidly than concentrating on verbal versions of the procedure.

7.3.3 Transgenerational history-taking

Whenever a client answers that she has had the problem or aspects of it "forever" or "ever since I can remember", it is a good idea to ask whether a parent has a similar problem and whether the client might have any idea about the source of the parent's stress. Often the problem experience can be traced back several generations, sometimes collective experiences (famines, wars, ethnic segregation, and persecution) can be identified as the origin of the problem, and sometimes it can be pinpointed to individual experiences such as the death of a child or an unhappy marriage several generations ago. Sometimes the origin remains obscure. The procedures in this section belong to the spectrum of therapeutic modelling.[6]

One option for dispelling stresses of this kind is to give them back to the people who experienced the symptoms first, or who triggered the symptoms in the client with their behaviour.

Bringing back symptoms (return style)

"Imagine that you could take all of this anxiety and uncertainty out of you and place it in front of you in a basket. What colour would the basket be? What kind of material would it be made of?

If your clone were to step out of you, take the basket and give whatever was in the basket back to whoever had given it to her, who would that be? Her father? Her mother? Someone else?

You can say to your father, 'There you go, father, I got this from you. It doesn't belong to me. I'm giving it back to you again. If you don't think it belongs to you either, give it back to the person you got it from. That person can pass it on as well if they like, but it's none of my business any more.' And you can say to your mother, 'There you go, mother, I'm giving this back to you. If you like, you can give it to the people you got it from, and they can pass it on …' How is that for you? How does that feel?"[7]

Dissociating ancestors (matryoshka style)

If it appears that the problem might have been passed down for generations, the mother can be taken out of her mother, and her mother out of her mother, etc. Another option is the method of genealogical division.

Dissociating ancestors (genealogical style)

"Imagine that your internal image of your father could step out of you, and we could place him over there. And we'll place the mother from out of your head over there.

Then we can take your father's father out of your father and place him just behind him, and your father's mother alongside him.

We'll take your mother's father and mother out of her, and put them a little behind her, to distinguish them from her.

Then we'll take your eight great-grandparents out of your four grandparents: great-grandfather, great-grandmother, great-grandfather, great-grandmother, great-grandfather, great-grandmother, great-grandfather, great-grandmother. Then your 16 great-great-grandparents out of your eight great-grandparents, and your 32 great-great-great-grandparents out of them and so on."

This procedure can be used repeatedly, with minor alterations. Another procedure that often allows clients and therapists to make extremely surprising discoveries reveals significant individual differences.

Liberating ancestors

"My eyes are no longer itchy, but my nose is still runny," said a woman at the start of her second session of therapy for a pollen allergy. I made further enquires about her symptoms, and asked her the following question.

"If the person who apparently still has some allergy left over and who has a runny nose were allowed to step out of you for once, where should she go and stand?"
"Over there."
"How does she look?"
"Oh!!! She's wearing a potato sack! That's odd!"
"Is she wearing a sack as if it were an item of clothing, or is she standing in it as though she were competing in a sack race?"
"She's wearing it as if it were an item of clothing."
"What colour hair does she have?"
"She's blond." (*The client has black hair.*)
"Then it's not you, it's someone else. How old is she?"
"Thirteen or fourteen. She's haggard and looks emaciated to the extreme. I think she's in a concentration camp." (*The client clears her throat.*)
"If the person who is clearing her throat also steps out of you, how does she look?"
"She has guilt issues. She's ashamed."
"Does that have anything to do with that girl over there?"
"Yes. She could have helped her, but didn't. She looked away. And I think the girl died."
"Is she a relative of yours?"
"I don't know."

"If she were a relative, would she be on your mother's or your father's side?"

"My mother's."

"Imagine if we were to take your image of your mother out of you, and put her over there … And then if we were to take out of your mother her own mother, and put her next to her … And then her mother next to her … So that your grandmother and great-grandmother are next to your mother … Would one of these women be the same as the one who is ashamed, or are they different?"

"I never knew my grandmother or great-grandmother, but my great-grandmother is the one who is ashamed."

"What was the connection between your great-grandmother and the haggard girl? Are they related?"

"I think the girl is her daughter. It must have been a teenage pregnancy – the way it used to be dealt with, where a girl would disappear for six months in order to finish the pregnancy in secret and then return without the baby."

"If you imagine that the most loving, warm-hearted and maternal person you can be steps out of you as a copy and goes over to the girl, hugs her, talks to her and tells her, 'Welcome to our family!', how does the girl react?"

"She's surprised. She says, 'I should have known all along that I belonged to you. Why did no one tell me that when I was alive?'"

"Did she not know who her mother was?"

"She suspected, but she wasn't certain."

"How does she look when she hears that?"

"She's happy that I've come to her, but she's sad and angry about what was done to her."

"If you say to her, 'How they treated you was awful. You didn't deserve that, not in the slightest. It was an appalling injustice. I'm sorry! I'd like to welcome you to our family, if I may!' how does she respond?"

"She smiles shyly."

"See what happens now if the loving person who you could be continues to hug her and talk to her … If we address your great-grandmother, who's guilty and ashamed, and say to her, 'The fact that you feel guilty and ashamed shows that you would have liked things to be different. It shows that you had love. You didn't manage to do what you would have deemed right. But you really do have love for your daughter,' how does she react?"

"She's now no longer looking at the ground. I believe she agrees with what you said."

"How does the girl react when she hears and sees that?"

"I think she's relieved. She just wishes that someone had told her that earlier."

"If the caring one over there calls over the one who was ashamed and hugs both, one in the left arm and one in the right, is that OK?"

"Yes, that's OK."

"And if she asks the mother and the daughter to look at each other and perhaps, if it feels right, also to hug each other, in a kind of group hug, how's that?"

"Good."

"And how's your nose now?"

"Better. Pretty good."

Bringing back symptoms (repossession style)

Rapid relief can be provided if the therapist says something along the lines of the following.

"That's terrible for your grandmother. But now it should be obvious that it's not your sadness. The sadness belongs to your grandmother. You can tell your grandmother, 'What you experienced was awful. But this sadness belongs to you, not me. I'd like to give it back to you again.' What does she say to that?"
"She accepts the sadness. She doesn't want me to have it."
"How do you feel now?"
"Much better."

Separating images of yourself and others (de-identification)

In response to the question, "Is this person who has been taken out you a version of you, or someone else?" a client might answer doubtfully,

"It's me – kind of – but somehow the person looks like a man."
"Let's turn it into two people: we'll place a version of you to the left, and a man on the right.[8] Do you have any idea who the man might be?"
"It's my father."

Separating emotional stresses (by causes)

The therapist might perceive something sad in the client's expression, and suggest the following: "If there is someone who is sad, can we place him next to you?" If the client then continues to look just as sad as before, the therapist can propose,

"Are there perhaps several of them who are sad?"
"Yes, perhaps."
"If we try putting them over there – how many of them are there?"
"Between ten and fifteen or thereabouts."
"Do they all look like you, or like someone else?"

Separating emotional stresses (by persons)

Sometimes a client will respond that they are all versions of herself, sometimes that they are all other people, and sometimes that some of them are versions of herself and some are other people. The therapist can continue as follows:

"How many of them are versions of you?"
"Wait a minute, just let me finish counting ... seven."
"And the others, are they men or women?"
"Some are men and some are women."

"Do you know them?"

"Yes, that's my father and my mother and my grandmother, my mother's mother, she's there twice. And then there's someone else, it might be my great-grandmother, my grandmother's mother. But I never met her."

Occasionally hundreds, or rarely even thousands or hundreds of thousands of sad, anxious, angry or lonely figures step out of a client; in such cases, these figures are predominantly not versions of the client herself. A phenomenon of this kind is sometimes to be observed in clients of Jewish or Armenian extraction, or whose family experienced particular stresses during wartime.

Asking persons to appear from behind a veil of silence

Based on my experience, if clients describe a person as transparent, a grey space, or faceless, these are people who died early, for example in the womb, or who are concealed behind a "veil of silence" by a family that pretends that they do not exist. In such cases it can be very interesting to direct a friendly request to the person perceived as "shadowy" to make themselves visible, whereupon the individual in question may well then appear front of the client's inner eye in a much more clearly recognisable form.

I cannot be sure of the extent to which the persons described by clients bear any relation to actual characters and events, unless clients refer to events that are in any case familiar to them from family stories. I am also unable to guess at the extent to which the nature of the question is a factor determining the figures that appear. All I can say is that neither my clients nor I are able to foresee any of what unfolds within a short space of time, and that even with hindsight I am unable to gauge what I might have contributed to the outcome apart from my questions, which were not aimed at exercising any substantive influence; it is of course clear that a therapist cannot ask anything without suggesting possible answers. It is also obvious that the vast majority of clients experience the outcomes that are identified or developed as intensely realistic and relevant to them.

I do not know whether these are family memories that have been stored (either epigenetically or in a kind of collective unconscious), fictions that align with the client's physical experience and social behaviour, or reconstructions or new constructions of an event that explains the client's experience. It is worth noting that dispelling the unhappiness of these figures by showing them respectful and empathic attention frequently helps to dispel the symptoms described in physical, mental, and social terms by the client.

Asking ancestors for absolution and blessing

One option for relieving burdens that are expressed in images of this kind is to ask the ancestors who represent the starting point of the unfortunate family tradition to absolve the client (and other ancestors, if applicable) from the duty to engage in the self-harming behaviour and experience that has been handed down over generations. This tradition can be interpreted as a contract or oath which, following an initial traumatic experience on the part of one ancestor, has been passed on to future generations, and which family members have sworn. The content of this vow can also be made explicit in the therapeutic conversation, in the following manner: "I solemnly vow that I will always do XYZ/never do XYZ – regardless of what it costs!" Wording the vow in this way obviously only makes sense if the vow is then dissolved with an equal sense of ceremony.[9]

A less formal approach is also possible. If the client reaches a conclusion (or an assumption that is perceived to be correct) about which of her ancestors was the first to experience this stress or perceived duty, she can imagine this person in front of her and enter into a dialogue with them. She can ask this person to absolve her from the burden of this legacy, and to give her a blessing so that she can live her life freely. (Another option is to ask the last ancestor who did not yet exhibit this behaviour to absolve the client.)

In response to the question of whether this person is willing to do what has been asked, clients typically say that the person is very happy to do so. It is only in very rare cases that clients report that the ancestor is hesitant. In these cases, it is usually possible to identify what is making the person hesitate or what the person needs by means of further questions. Acknowledging their burden, valuing their good intentions, rephrasing the blessing that has been asked for or addressing another specific ancestor typically then leads to the desired outcome. The therapist can ask the following questions.

"If you imagine your ancestor saying to you, 'I absolve you from the burden of this legacy and give you my blessing to live your life free from this stress!', how does he look while he is saying this? How does that feel?" If necessary, the therapist can suggest that the client should imagine saying these words from the ancestor's perspective, while at the same time experiencing the internal attitude with which the ancestor says them (perhaps strength, love, and truthfulness) – and that she should then return to her previous perspective as the client, and allow the words she has spoken and heard to reverberate within her. The therapist can also ask her the following questions.

"Does it matter what your ancestor says? Would you like to put yourself over there and say that, and experience how it feels to stand there in that place and to say that to the you who is sitting here? Or do we not even need to bother doing that?"

A ritual of this kind can make a lasting contribution to helping people to leave behind them the symptoms described in physical, mental, and social terms that have accompanied them their whole life long, and even affected previous generations.

7.3.4 Additive history-taking

The method of therapeutic modelling is also a viable option if one wishes to transition from taking the history of problems to taking the history of resources. By exploring what the objective looks like using hypothetical questions, the therapist is already laying the ground for the objective to be achieved in the client's imagination.

The therapist can then address the client, who might have described herself as fearful, indecisive, and self-accusing, by placing opposite her the "target person" she can be once she has overcome her problem.

"Supposing that the person who you are when you look into the world with optimism, certainty, love, and self-confidence, when you enjoy looking at yourself in the mirror, when you love yourself and experience yourself as deeply loved – regardless of where the person you're imagining you are gets it from – came out of the world of possibilities, and is now standing over there, What is her posture like? How does she look? How is she breathing?"

"What might this beautiful, strong, self-confident person you're imagining you are say to you if you tell her about the difficulties you just told me about?"

Perhaps the client will express the belief that this person does not think she is someone worth talking to. This would suggest that she has not developed in the direction of this person up until now because she believes that people like that are arrogant or would be regarded as arrogant within her family (or in other words her community of values) and excluded from the community. In order to experience a sense of belonging within this community, it might seem safer to her not to become like this person. The therapist could drill down into this subject as follows.

"I imagine that she'd be able to listen to you with empathy and compassion, and that she'd be a good and respectful listener. And precisely because she's self-aware, she doesn't need to look down on others – what do you think?"

The conversation can then turn to the matter of trying out how it would be to experience both at the same time: being as optimistic and self-confident as this person, and experiencing a sense of belonging to one's own family and loyalty to their system of values.

If a client would like to lose weight, the therapist can ask the following questions.

"Supposing that the person who you are when you weigh five kilograms less is sitting here, how does she look? How do you think she feels? What else sets her apart?"

When discussing the target experience, it might be the case that the client says something like, "She feels vulnerable and a bit exposed."

The therapist can ask the client if she has any ideas about the background to this experience. In the process, he'll learn about the latent factors that have prevented the client from losing weight for good up until now. Perhaps the client will talk about a period during which she did in fact weigh five kilograms less, but which was a very difficult time in her life. Maybe she will talk about how she previously suffered from anorexia, about her first boyfriend and the break-up with him, and about how she swore back then that she would never be thin again.

Memories and fears that run counter to the objective can thus be identified on the basis of the discomfort or scepticism associated with its image. The therapist can examine each of these life experiences and beliefs individually in order to take away from them the experience of relevance and plausibility in terms of interpreting the client's future life.

The therapist will undoubtedly also ask the client to experiment with how it might be possible and how it would feel to weigh five kilograms less while at the same time feeling protected and safe.

Notes

1 See Chapter 8, section "Therapeutic maps and landscapes"/"The mountain village".
2 Ibid., section "Therapeutic spaces"/"Circle models".
3 Ibid., section "Therapeutic rituals"/"Healing rituals".
4 For further details of work with clients who come to therapy unwillingly, see Schmidt 2005, 106 *et seq.*
5 See Chapter 8, section "Therapeutic greetings".
6 See Chapter 2, section on psychodrama, constellation work and parts work as well as Chapter 8, section "Therapeutic modelling". A detailed description of therapeutic modelling can be found in Hammel 2019b.
7 See Hammel 2014a, 124 *et seqq.*
8 Or vice versa – left and right are referred to only as a means of generating a vivid image which can be used again by the therapist and client if necessary.
9 The procedure of asking an ancestor to absolve an individual from a family duty can be traced back to shamanic traditions. The Canadian therapist Sarah Peyton has linked the procedure to constellation work and a request for a blessing, see Peyton 2021, xi, 23 *et seq.* Following the discovery that many of the symptomatic people who are "taken out of" the client during therapeutic modelling are identified by these clients as very specific ancestors, I have taken to initiating simple dialogues between clients and these ancestors on the topic of "absolution and blessing". When doing so, I have observed the same immensely freeing effects reported by Sarah Peyton.

Chapter 8

Forms of therapeutic intervention

This chapter contains interventions that are aimed not at greeting a client, clarifying her objective, or taking her history, but simply at the therapy itself.

Of course, it is impossible to rule out entirely the possibility that therapy will also revert back to the taking of a more detailed history or a further clarification of objectives, because the client's experience has changed so much that new horizons loom into view ...

8.1 Therapeutic metaphors

Working with metaphors can be helpful when characterising problems that have been experienced. The process of establishing clarity that takes place at the same time, almost incidentally, can be used as a basis for transitioning smoothly into a process of healing. Clients may find metaphorical interventions surprising. Sometimes it can be a good idea to introduce the metaphors in such a way as to make it clear that this unconventional approach has specifically been chosen to provide the client with particular assistance with her issue. Often a sentence or phrase suffices, as follows.

"If I imagine what you're saying in very visual terms, I see before me ..."
"You're 'under pressure' ... If I were to take that expression literally, I could imagine ..."
"Sometimes I come up with slightly odd ideas. I hope that's OK with you. I imagine to myself ..."

Client feedback on the use of metaphors of this kind is exceptionally positive, even in the absence of introductory sentences of this kind. The following sections provide examples of the different types of therapeutic metaphors. There are an infinite number of other options for structuring metaphors in addition to the categories proposed here.

8.1.1 Order

Particularly during the first phase of therapy, when the client is describing his problems, metaphors can be used effectively in keeping with the rule of "separate

DOI: 10.4324/9781003425014-11

problems, link solutions". This approach has impressive effects. People who describe themselves as hopeless, overburdened, and paralysed at the start of a therapy session can develop a remarkably powerful and optimistic attitude within as little as 20 or 30 minutes. The creation of a "filing cabinet for problems" is an example of how this approach can be used systematically.[1]

The filing cabinet

The therapist can invite his client to imagine a filing cabinet in which she can file all of her problems. It goes without saying that the drawers should also be labelled so that the problems can be retrieved if they are ever needed again. The peculiar thing about filing cabinets is that it is only ever possible to open one drawer at a time, or to keep them all closed. The therapist can ask the client to imagine the filing cabinet and then mime the action of filling up its drawers himself, or he can visualise the cabinet and its drawers on a flipchart, a notepad or (during video calls) a digital whiteboard. He can then open each of the drawers one by one with the client, work together with the client to label them, and fill them up with all the problems that belong in that particular drawer.

"What will you write on the first drawer?"
"My relationship."
"So we'll fill up the first drawer with everything that stresses you out about your
    relationship ..."

Strictly speaking, this is minimal reframing rather than mirroring. I recommend putting the stresses that result from the relationship in the drawer rather than the relationship itself, and certainly not the client's partner.

"... There we go, now the drawer's open! In goes all of the irritation! In go the
    worries! In goes the fear! In goes the loneliness you feel! In goes the anger! In
    goes any sorrow there might be! In go the feelings of guilt! In go any feelings
    of shame there might be! In go all the disagreeable memories! In go all the
    negative expectations! In go all the hostile thoughts! In go the insults and hurts!
    Anything else?"
"I think that's probably about it ..."
"In goes everything that we might perhaps have forgotten! And now let's close the
    drawer!"
"What are you going to write on the next drawer?"
"Work-related stress."
"Right then! Let's open the drawer! You can add a number of different suspension
    files to separate the different problems from each other. Now let's get started!
    In goes the stress caused by your colleagues! In goes the stress caused by your
    boss! In goes all the stress caused by customers! In goes the stress caused by
    business partners, the authorities, anyone else who might be involved, the stress

caused by your own high standards … If anything I say is not quite right, adapt it so that it fits better! Anything else?"

"The boss's girlfriend who has just started working in the business as well …"

"In goes the stress caused by the boss's partner. Anything else?"

"I think that's it."

At the end, the therapist can create a "Miscellaneous" drawer for everything the client hasn't thought of or doesn't want to talk about right now.

If the therapist wants to, he can also move onto a second stage in which he asks the client about her favourite resources. What does she particularly like doing? What are some of her favourite memories? What can she do particularly well? He can then jot down a word or two for each resource in the space next to the filing cabinet. He can reach an agreement with the client that she should place a copy of one or more of these experiences into each drawer so that the feeling associated with these good life experiences is always there too, and perhaps, whenever the drawer is opened again later, they can even drown out with their sounds or smells the problems that have been stored away. The therapist can then open each drawer again together with the client, and place a resource inside ("The birth of my daughter", etc.). He can make a note of which resource is in which drawer by assigning a letter or number to them (Figure 8.1).

Clients can often be observed letting out a deep breath as they close each drawer, and then seeming more relaxed. When asked whether anything is different after filling up the filing cabinet (or whether we might just as well get the things back out again), they typically respond with a reference to positive changes. This improvement is frequently also observable during the next session,

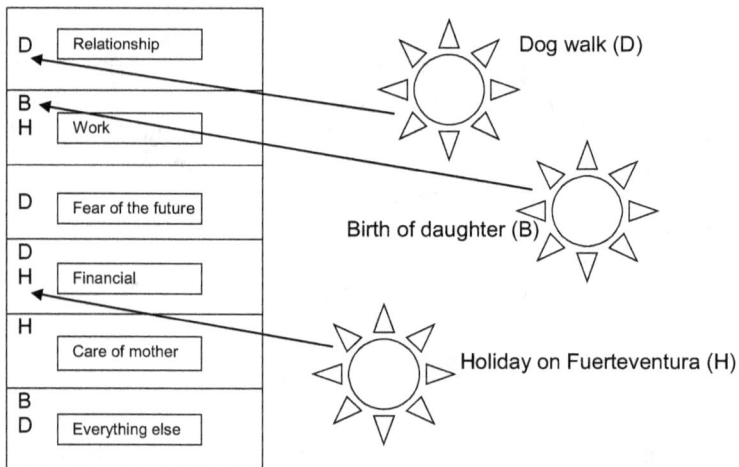

Figure 8.1 The filing cabinet

particularly in the case of clients with a variety of different stresses or depressive tendencies.

The image of the filing cabinet can be returned to in later sessions if need be, but this is not absolutely necessary in order for this way of working to be effective.[2]

8.1.2 Regulation

Physical, mental, and social symptoms can be interpreted as clues to "misunderstandings in the system". Hyperfunctions, hypofunctions, or malfunctions occur because various parts of the system, or in other words the body, self-image, family, or society, do not respond favourably to one another or to challenges from the exterior. This means that something is done too much, too little, or in a manner that is qualitatively different to what is needed. The body must therefore be stimulated in order to carry out the necessary adjustments at a later point in time. For example, many clients find it easy to regulate physical and mental functions if they think of appliances that are used to regulate certain physical variables.

Turning the heating up or down

I presented the following metaphor to a woman who had come to therapy and who suffered from Raynaud's syndrome (a circulatory disorder).[3]

"Supposing that it was a very harsh winter and you were freezing cold, even though all the radiators were supposed to be on – you'd probably go and turn up the thermostat for the central heating system. If you weren't sure how to do it because you'd just moved in, you'd find someone who might know. Now imagine going on a walk on a very cold winter's day, and notice what changes in your hands, fingers, toes, and your whole body during the walk. Your body can ask someone who knows their way around the heating system inside you to repair the heating pipes, bleed the radiators, and turn up the thermostat so that all of the rooms get warm."[4]

Metaphors of this kind can also be staged as a therapeutic ritual during the session or as a task to be completed at home.[5]

The brake cable

When working with a woman who could hardly move her thumb due to carpal tunnel syndrome, I spoke about the problematic bodily function as follows.

"Tendons have a sheath, and they move around in this sheath just like a bicycle brake cable moves around in its tubing. Imagine pulling the brake cable out of the tubing, sanding it down until it shines, oiling it and stretching and dilating the tubing until the cable moves smoothly inside it. Now stretch and move your thumb again ..."

The woman managed to complete the movement effortlessly. When I asked several weeks later, and again several years later, she said that she had repeated "the thing with the brake cable" several times herself in the weeks following our conversation. In the process the issue had vanished and had not reappeared.[6] I have carried out the intervention with several other clients, almost always with the same outcome.

Sound engineer and mixing desk

It is possible to work with clients experiencing the symptoms of tinnitus using the metaphor of a sound engineer who is mixing a track for a band at his mixing desk. He can make the sound levels of the different microphones louder, quieter, or even silent, and he can adjust the balance of bass and treble to very different levels with reference to the different frequencies. The metaphor can also be used for people with auditory processing problems and for those who experience noises as emotionally stressful (hyperacusis, those subjected to snoring, misophonia).

It often proves challenging to try and reduce the overall volume of tinnitus. In the case of many clients, it has turned out that the various partial noises are associated with different biographical stresses, which apparently want to be addressed in different ways. I have found that a useful approach in these cases is to divide the tinnitus up into partial noises or frequencies, and to allow the client to experiment with which noise goes quiet first, which second etc.

For some clients it might be advisable to make the noises somewhat louder to begin with, and only then to make them quieter. Certain people find it easier to develop an expectation that the noises can become quieter once they have realised that they have the power to make them louder. What is more, this test is also valuable in terms of therapeutic history-taking; if a client can make the noise louder but not quieter, his internal self definitely knows how to regulate the volume, but is effectively imposing a veto.

When I asked one client what his internal self might have against the sound disappearing, she answered, "Then I'd have to face up to the issues that relate to my work, and then I wouldn't be able to work any more." A few days later her tinnitus disappeared, and the mental stress resulting from her work became so great that she took sick leave and considered retirement. She came to the conclusion that she and her husband had hardly spent any time together for many years, and that her marriage therefore had little chance of lasting the course. They decided to make their relationship a conscious priority and to stay together. A few weeks later she moved to a new job. The tinnitus came back, but she reported that the volume was much lower and she found it significantly less stressful in emotional terms.

8.1.3 Equilibrium

Many stresses can be interpreted as indicating that something has come out of equilibrium.

People with compulsions pursue a value such as hygiene or safety, or avoiding violence, religious impurity or sin, so strenuously that other values such as self-preservation, a zest for life, and efficiency at work are neglected and then make space for themselves impulsively.

It is possible that individuals with eating disorders and addictive tendencies are attempting to reduce their suffering (loneliness, grief, humiliation etc.) using substances, activities, and media that numb their pain at the same time as bringing about undesirable side effects.

Metaphors can help clients to live in an equilibrium of values instead of putting individual values into practice at the expense of others. I might explain something along the lines of the following to clients with compulsive thoughts or compulsive actions, or to others who are suffering from the symptoms of burnout and exhaustion.

The fight on the barricades

Only people with strong values can experience compulsion. If you wish to put a value into practice wholeheartedly, for example non-aggression, another value – such as self-preservation or self-respect – will be neglected. In turn, this value will find it unfair if others take advantage of you simply because you are generous. Perhaps it will also find it concerning that you take advantage of yourself on behalf of others who do not thank you for it. Your self-preservation will make ructions and take to the barricades. The more the "values police" now attempts to suppress and control these impulses, the more self-preservation will fight for its right to have space of its own, to be treated just as well as the others and to defend itself against injustice if necessary. And the more it defends itself, the more the "values police" will try and suppress the uprising. It's not at all easy to say who's right. Struggles of this kind can go on for a long time. It is better to invite both sides to sit at the same table: the representatives of friendliness and the representatives of self-preservation and self-respect. After all, both sides represent values! During mediation, the positive values, legitimate needs, and positive intentions of both sides can be mapped out, followed by a process of finding out how the good that both sides want can be achieved in a mutual equilibrium. This is not a simple "compromise": it is entirely possible that afterwards the values on both sides will be able to perform their tasks better than before.[7]

Foxes and hares

"Anyone who experiences compulsion is thorough and loves to implement certain values to the absolute max. Frugality can be a value, and so can generosity.

Willpower is a value, and so is flexibility. Yet anyone who is frugal to the max cannot be generous to the max; anyone has an eye on the bigger picture cannot concentrate on what really matters, and vice versa! What is to be done in such a situation?

Give a greeting to the person in your brain who is thorough and loves perfection; ask her to continue with her work, but from now on to optimise values instead of maximising them. That's something completely different. Let me explain what I mean.

Imagine you're a forest ranger who's responsible for a large forest, and so you're interested in the health of this forest. When is a forest healthy? You might say, 'When as many foxes as possible are living there,' but then there wouldn't be many hares, and so soon the number of foxes would decline. You might also say, 'When as many hares as possible are living there,' but then they'd strip everything bare. If there's lots of wolves, there's no deer, but if there's lots of deer, there's no young trees. A good ecological balance can't be achieved by aiming for a maximum of any one thing.

You're much more likely to get a healthy forest if you say, 'I want as many individuals of as many different plant and animal species as possible, or in other words for the product of the number of species and the average number of individuals per species to be as large as possible.'

Optimising values means that the product of Value A times Value B times Value C times Value D is large because no value is a maximum – and therefore no value is a minimum. To put it another way, you'd have a relatively large amount of generosity at the same time as a relatively large amount of frugality, a good amount of willpower and a good amount of flexibility … Give a greeting to the previous 'maximiser' in you – do you think she's ready to become the best 'overall value optimiser' of all time on your behalf?"

8.1.4 Transfer

A "transfer" involves conveying information from one area to another. We can often also talk about "learning by example". Yet information is not passed on only between humans. It is also conveyed and evaluated non-verbally, or in other words between sub-functions of the body, between animals, plants, or also microorganisms, within one species and also between different species. Information is passed on using electrical systems, computers, or quantum mechanics, exchanged between cultures and organisations, handed on from one generation to the next, or created for the first time. What matters in our context is linking up authorities that have certain resources with those who require these resources, in order to transfer helpful information without it going astray at the place where it has so far been held.

The conference between the right and the left

In the case of symptoms that affect half or one side of the body, a conference can be convened between the right and the left. The procedure is similar to the intervention

"Instructor and pupil (utilisation of previous successes)".[8] This is a useful option in the case of injuries, hemiplegia, and functional deficiencies (strokes, multiple sclerosis), renal insufficiency and infections, for example, or, as in the following case, tinnitus.

> How does your quiet ear manage to hear silence? If the people from your body hold a conference between the right and the left and meet in working groups at this conference, those from one ear can show those from the other ear how the silence can be heard. Perhaps they notice that the muscular tension is not quite the same on the two sides of the face and perhaps even on the two sides of the body as a whole, or that it is exactly the same but needs to be different, or that the auditory cortex on the right of the brain works differently to that on the left and that the two need to be adjusted differently, or that they are already adjusted differently and it would be much better for them to be adjusted the same. Perhaps they notice that one side has a slight hearing impairment at certain frequencies that is absent from the other side, and that because of this slight hearing impairment the brain wants to set the low volume differently at certain frequencies than at others. What do the people from one side of the body, where there's still something to learn, learn from those on the other, and how do the people convey it to them in such a way that they can take it on board?[9]

Change of operating system

A student who had experienced a psychotic episode told me what I should say to people like him in relation to their remaining symptoms (their residual state):

> The change from psychosis to a normal state is like the change between two operating systems, for example Windows and Linux … It's possible that the programs and functions might not all run perfectly on the new operating system. The computer should scan the hard drive and replace or supplement the relevant parts as necessary.[10]

8.2 Therapeutic stories

Since we all involuntarily process our memories, expectations, and creative interpretations of the world in the form of night-time and day-time dreams, we continuously construct our life experiences as stories.[11] Dreams (or in other words figurative thoughts) could be interpreted as the body's mother tongue or as the primeval way of orienting oneself. This would make verbal language a coding and decoding system that allows dreams of this kind to be communicated so that the listener experiences them too.

Like any kind of invented or experienced stories, our day-time and night-time dreams can be subdivided into different types based on their structure. A distinction can be made between paradigmatic and metaphorical dreams, as well as between those with a happy, unhappy, and mysterious or open ending.

	Paradigm (anecdote, realistic scene)	Metaphor (parable, scene with figurative meaning)
Positive learning model	Dream about flirting Story with a happy ending	Dream about flying Living life like an eagle
Negative learning model	Dream about an argument Nightmare, tragedy	Dream about escaping Ending up like a sacrificial lamb
Searching model	Realistic puzzles Childhood friends: Are they still alive? Are they happy?	Metaphorical puzzles You open the treasure chest – look inside: what's there?

Where is it best for therapeutic stories to start, and where should the end goal be? That's a matter of pacing and leading. Life has ups and downs. The people who come to therapy are those who have experienced one of its downward turns, and are afraid that the situation will remain like that or get even worse. The purpose of therapy is to develop internal films that start with the client's initial experience and guide her to a better experience in viable steps.

Helpful internal films are stories that …

- are associatively based on her stressful experience so that she experiences them as relevant, and
- guide her away from her "memory" and "expectation" stories, so that she finds new ways of dealing with her challenges without entering into the previous states of pain and paralysis.

The therapist and the client develop stories that are analogous to the problem experience that has been described. These stories lead from a crisis to a solution, while at the same time leaving plenty of space for the client's own interpretations and for transfers. This prevents them from having a didactic or moralising effect. They are either developed spontaneously based on the conversation[12] or prepared in between sessions.[13]

The protagonist of the story can be the client herself, who is reminded of previous crises that were overcome, the therapist, or another real or fictitious person. Fictitious persons can take either a realistic or an infinite number of fantastic forms. The route from the problem to the solution is "perceived to be plausible", or in other words the rules of the genre are observed: fairy tales involve someone doing magic, fables involve talking animals, and scientific and biographical accounts involve neither of these things.

The situation can be illustrated as shown in Figure 8.2.

1. A client reaches a low point in the story of her life due to stressful events (*dark-grey circle in centre of diagram representing life's ups and downs*) and goes to counselling.

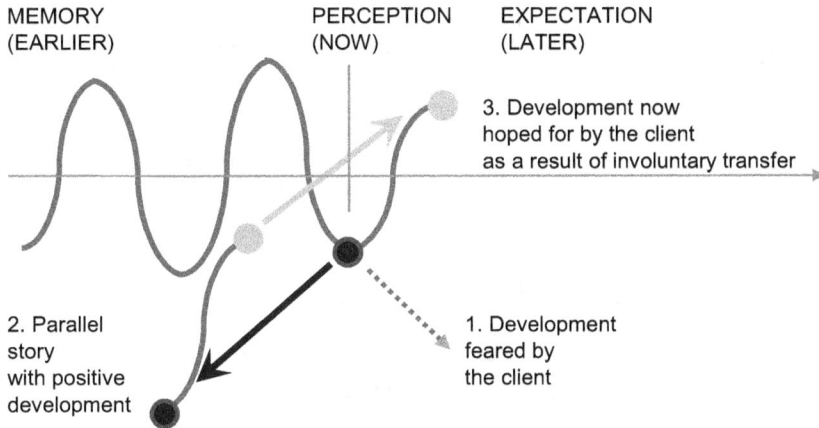

Figure 8.2 Creating positive expectation by dropping a story starting bad and turning positive

2. The therapist presents to him a parallel story that develops plausibly from a low point (*dark-grey circle on diagram, bottom left*) to a high point (*light-grey circle near centre of diagram*).
3. By consciously following this story and accepting it, the client involuntarily starts to use the story's positive course as a basis for predicting her own story (*light-grey circle on diagram, top right*).

In order to develop a story with a plot and a coherent ending spontaneously, or indeed to do so without any rush between two therapy sessions, it is sufficient to remember the following six sentences or the words printed in bold in the correct order. This script can be used to structure fables, anecdotes, stories from the therapist's own life, and any number of invented or "true" stories as a *positive learning model*.

1. Introduce the **protagonist** (animal, child, an acquaintance, myself) and his world.
2. Describe the protagonist's **problem**.
3. List unsuccessful **attempted solutions** (at the location or on a journey to the solution).
4. **Failure**: exhibit frustration, perplexity, sadness (each time or once on a cumulative basis)!
5. An external or internal mentor facilitates **ideas**, discovery, homecoming.
6. Celebrate **success**.

"Doctor Badger" is an example of this approach.[14]

If the outcome is to remain open in order to provoke further contemplation (**searching model**), the story can end at Point 5 in a question or a mysterious plot twist that triggers an internal search.

The client tells life stories
from low point to low point ...

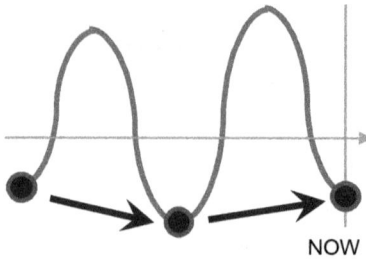

... and the therapist mirrors them as
stories from high point to high point.

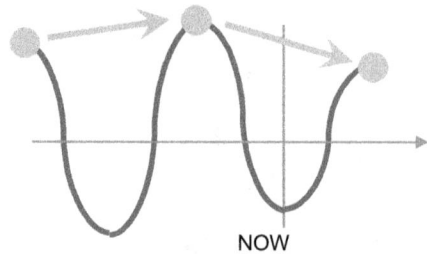

NOW   NOW

Figure 8.3 Telling life stories from low point to low point or from high point to
high point

Or: the client presents the story
from high point to low point ...   ...and the therapist mirrors it as a story
from low point to high point.

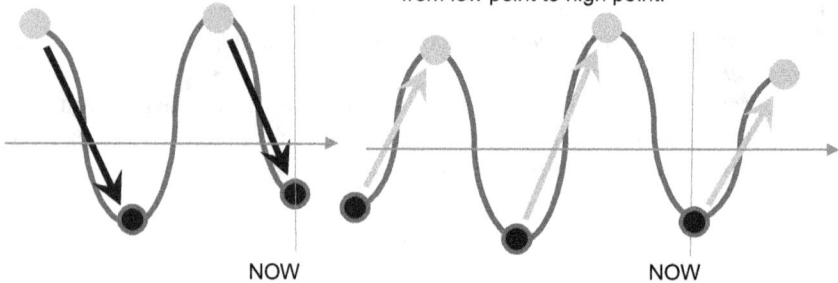

NOW   NOW

Figure 8.4 Telling life stories from high point to low point or from low point to
high point

A catastrophic ending after Point 4 (*negative learning model*) is another potential
option. It should, however, be noted that this is only therapeutically appropriate if the
client does not see herself as failing, if she manifestly has enough resources to deal
with her situation, and if the ending does not have a didactic, derogatory, or moralising effect. This calls for tact, and is most likely to succeed if the story is presented as
a humorous challenge among friends or if it has more of a metaphorical bent.[15]

Another narrative category involves changing the punctuation of the stories told
by the client, or in other words retelling the client's life story in a respectful manner
by relocating the starting and ending points of the different sections of the story
(Figures 8.3 and 8.4).[16]

If we take a closer look at the trajectory shown at the start, all of these various
models of punctuation are entirely admissible. In terms of the client's well-being,
however, the punctuation options shown on the right are more likely to be more
beneficial than those on the left.

8.2.1 Altered punctuation

Various options for altering punctuation in terms of the chronology of events are set out below.

Betrayed four times (from low point to high point)

A woman said to me, "I've had cancer four times. My body betrayed me four times!" "You've recovered four times. Your body healed you four times." "But it was the doctors who did that!" "It was your body that did that. Doctors can't heal you. They can only help your body to heal itself." "Do you think so? Is that what you believe?" "Yes, that's exactly what I believe!"

The child that almost suffocated (from high point to high point)

"Perhaps the problem is that I spoil my son too much," said the woman who was sitting in front of me. Next to her sat her 20-year-old son, whom she was worried about because he was so passive, and her ex-husband. "That's because he almost died when he was born." "How did that happen?" I enquired. "Just after David was born – while I was still recovering – my husband took him out into the hospital garden and sat down on a bench. Then he fell asleep, but in a position that meant that the air was being squeezed out of David. He was already turning blue. A doctor who happened to be passing by tore the baby out of his arms and rushed him off to the NICU." The young man next to her – the baby from back then – looked healthy and cheerful. I asked the woman to keep on telling me her story … and so we continued for a while. To begin with her voice was hesitant, but as she reached the point where they all came home in good health, it sounded warm and fluent. "I can understand why you've ended the story in the NICU every time that you've told it up until now," I said. "It's likely that you freeze at this point whenever you tell the story, just like back then when you learned what had happened in the garden. But that wasn't the ending – this right here is the real ending of the story. I'd like to ask you to tell yourself this story out loud another five times when you're back at home, and to make sure that you continue all the way up to this point every time."

Encounter in heaven (from high point to high point in spite of a catastrophe)

"But what if the child had died?" I was asked by a participant in a seminar. "Surely the story wouldn't have a happy ending then! "If the child had died, there will be no happy ending on earth. So I'd look even further into the future. I'd ask the woman, 'If you imagine that there's a heaven and your child is there, and if you imagine that you visit your son there – how does he greet you? How does he look at you?' I'd enquire how the greeting in heaven would go: 'If you explain to him what is bothering you: grief, feelings of guilt, criticism of your husband … What will you tell him? What will he answer in return? Does he mean it? Does that sound right? How do you feel about that?'"

In my experience, the dead are merciful. What they say is typically wise and generous. Following an encounter of this kind, I remind the mother that this particular journey can be followed by many more, and that mother and child can keep on meeting each other frequently in this manner. The child can also travel down from heaven and visit the therapy room. The effect is the same.

8.2.2 Shared life experience

We can use stories that draw upon the client's own life stories to say something about the current problem experience that we hope to transform into a resource and solution experience. We can choose stories leading from minor crises to major successes, or from major crises to surprising solutions. Below are examples of each of these two alternatives.

Instructor and pupil (utilisation of previous successes)

I asked a young man with tinnitus who had come to therapy about his hobbies and interests.

"Do you do any sport?" "Taekwondo." "Which belt?" "Second dan." If the young man had been an ice skater, Formula 1 driver, or sports marksman, I would have asked him about that sport, and the effect would have been the same. I said, "Listen to me. Imagine that your left ear, which is an expert at silence, is the instructor. Your right ear, which is familiar with tinnitus, is the pupil. What can the instructor teach the pupil, and what would the pupil like to learn from his instructor?" "Concentration." "Good. Listen to the instructor for a while as he teaches his pupil. Watch the pupil listening to his instructor and doing what he says." A few minutes later, the young man turned to me: "Now everything is quiet."[17]

You'll be able to do it when it matters (utilisation of previous crises)

We can also remind the client of major crises she has overcome. In keeping with the rule that a certain amount of transfer work should be left to the client in order to avoid seeming patronising, didactic, or moralising, it is often a better idea to choose examples that are a long way from the client's initial situation instead of those closer at hand.

Some time ago, a colleague's daughter complained that she had problems with her memory. "If I need to know ten answers to an exam question, I can normally only remember five or six." "Are you sure that it's always the same five or six answers?" asked her mother. "Or do you perhaps remember different answers every time, and so you do actually know all the answers in general?" "I think it's different answers I can't remember each time. Perhaps I do know them all in general. But what good does that do me? There's still some missing every time." "I agree that you know all the answers in general. And so you'll remember all of them in the exam when it really matters. Right now it doesn't really matter, and so your brain knows that you don't need to come up with all the answers, and only gives you some of them. But in the exam your brain will tell you all the answers." "And how do I know that?" "Remember when we were mugged on holiday in Colombia? Back then you ran faster than you'd ever run in your whole life. And afterwards you said, 'I didn't know that I could run so fast.' You could run that fast because you needed to. You hadn't needed to beforehand, and that's why you hadn't been able to. Exactly the same is true for what you've revised and your exam." The daughter appeared reassured and carried on revising. She passed the exam and remembered all of the answers.[18]

8.2.3 Role models

The life experiences of famous and less famous people can be used as models for successful solutions – or as a model of what not to do. The "Guggenheim" intervention is a positive learning model, and "Barbarossa" is an example of a negative learning model. The "happy ending" here is that the client does it differently to the protagonist ...

Meet me at the Guggenheim

At a meeting of artists, a photographer shared photos of an exhibition he had held in the famous Guggenheim Museum.

"How on earth did you manage to get an exhibition there?" he was asked by a friend.

"I sent in an application in 2010. They didn't respond. Then I sent in an application in 2011. They refused. Then I sent in an application in 2012. That didn't work either. Then I applied in 2013. They didn't want me then either. Then I applied again in 2014. That time they said 'yes'. Keep at it, that's all that matters."

Barbarossa

I use this story particularly for people suffering from physical tension, pain, physical rigidity, hyposensitivity, alexithymia, and various dissociative phenomena, presumably as a result of previous trauma. The process is based on the therapeutic principle of making paralysed emotions perceptible without them taking over.[19] It is worth acting out the story in the form of a mime in order to make it even more readily accessible to the senses. It can also be turned into an intervention similar to the healing ritual, "Pulling symptoms out of the body".[20]

"Once upon a time, a very long time ago, Emperor Barbarossa was returning from a crusade. All the fighting was over and done with, but he kept his armour on during the long journey home as a precaution. After all, you never know.

They came to a point where they had to cross a river. They found a ford where the horses would manage to get across. Yet in the middle of the river it so happened that Barbarossa's horse lost his footing. The Emperor fell, and since his armour was so heavy, he drowned. The country entered a period of deep mourning, and even today some people say that he didn't drown, but simply went into hiding.

"When a war is over, it's a good idea to take off your armour: first the helmet with the visor. Place it in front of you, and see how it looks ... Then the breastplate. Look at that too ... Now the backplate. See ... The upper arm pieces on the right and left ... The lower arm pieces ... The gauntlets with their delicate hinges ... The upper leg pieces ... The lower leg pieces ... The sabatons ... Is there anything missing? Of course! Next comes the chain mail ... Where are you going to put it? ... And then the leather doublet under the chain mail ... Is that going next to the chain mail, or should we hang it over this chair here? ... Is that everything, or is there anything else you can remove? ... Now ask your man-at-arms to take it all and place it in the arsenal. And ask your valet to bring your imperial robes. Would you like to dress yourself, or would you like to be dressed by him?"

We can also draw on our own experiences, provided that the client is not left with the impression that we are pushing the client's concerns to one side or somehow profiting at her expense. It is a good idea to make it clear in such cases that we are aware of what the client is suffering, instead of focusing on how good we feel now that the situation has been resolved.

You can do it!

On 19 June 1974, my old class teacher was writing reports. In my report she wrote the following: "Stefan's accomplishments are satisfactory. However he could achieve much more if he did not suffer from a severe behavioural disorder. He is completely incapable of concentrating, lacks self-confidence and often seems tense and scared. He needs to work in a more orderly fashion."

On 16 June 2008, I was speaking to eight children in a psychiatric outpatients' clinic: "When I was as old as you are now, I had almost no friends. The other children tormented me and laughed at me. My teacher wrote in my report: 'He will fail because of his inability to work quickly and his behavioural problems.' She was wrong. I succeeded in life. You will too."[21]

The therapist can also incorporate his own experiences in the third person. (Erickson used the pseudonym "my friend John" in such cases.) Similarly, the experiences of other clients, friends, and family members can also be used provided that care is taken to ensure that the persons referred to cannot be identified.

8.2.4 Fairy tales, fables, fantasy stories

The six-step rule has proven effective when developing fantasy stories. In terms of plot, it is important to make it clear that the problem is not trivial and that the development of a solution is challenging but possible. The fable of "Doctor Badger" can be used to reduce the fear of medical treatment in children (e.g. a phobia of needles) or to induce a mental anaesthesia (active–alert hypnosis). It can furthermore serve as an example illustrating the six-step schema of traditional therapeutic stories.

Doctor Badger

1. **Introduce the protagonist:** The fox had stepped on a thorn.
2. **Describe the problem:** It was deep in his paw, and walking on that paw hurt terribly.
3. **List the attempted solutions:** Soon the fox was running around on only three paws. He kept the fourth raised up in the air, which did indeed mean that it didn't hurt much. But of course that wasn't very practical, and he also couldn't chase hares like that.

The other animals shook their heads and said, "Go to the badger, perhaps he can help you." The badger played the role of doctor to the other animals. He knew what needed to be done if one of them was ill or had injured themselves. The badger examined the fox's paw closely and said, "There's a thorn in there. There's no two ways about it, we'll need to get it out." But as soon as the badger began to pull on the thorn, the fox whipped his paw away and gave a terrible cry, because now it had really started to hurt. "You're hurting me!" said the fox. "I have to pull on the thorn so that it comes out," said the badger. "It might hurt a lot, but the pain will only last a short time."

4. **Outline a failure:** The two could not agree, and so the fox continued to hobble around through the forest on three legs for another few days, getting more and more hungry.
5. **Present a new idea:** "Can't you think of another way of getting it out?" he asked the badger when he saw him again. "Come with me!" replied the badger, and together they went down to the river. "Hold your paw in there. The water's so cold that it will numb your paw." The fox stretched out his paw and placed it in the water. "Brrr! That's cold!" It was very unpleasant, but the badger was right. After a while he could barely feel his paw any more. "What are you doing this evening?" asked the badger. The fox thought for a while.
6. **Celebrate success:** While he was thinking, the badger took his paw, pulled on the thorn, and out it came.[22]

8.3 Therapeutic maps and landscapes

Presenting therapeutic situations as maps or landscapes can be an effective way of helping to lead clients or client systems out of a problem trance. A number of possibilities are presented in this section.

8.3.1 *The Island of Love*

The "Island of Love" map (Figure 8.5) is a good way of helping couples to discuss conflicts in a less acrimonious and harsh manner, and of moving the discussion onto a new level: "I've noticed that you sometimes live out your conflicts very intensely. If you'd just like to have a quick look at this map ..." The couple are immediately distracted from discussing their problems, and focused on something creative.

The therapist can continue with circular questions, as follows: "If I were to ask your husband where he's spent most of his time on this island recently (while things were so difficult), what do you think he would answer?" The client might say, "On the Cliffs of Failure." The therapist can then turn to the husband: "And if I were to ask your wife where she's spent most of her time during this period, what do you think she would say?" The client might say, "At the River of Tears."

The therapist can use different-coloured playing pieces to mark both locations.

Then he can address the husband and wife in turn as follows. "If I'd asked you directly, what would you have said?" He should then note down their answers. If the locations where they each believed the other would be are close to the locations where they situated themselves, the therapist can say, "You know each other well, and you're aware of how the other is feeling – that's a great starting point for our work." If the locations are a long way apart from each other, he can say, "The two of you have very different ideas about your respective locations. It's hardly surprising that you misunderstand each other. What we'll do now is try to align your ideas about yourselves and about each other so that these misunderstandings are no longer necessary."

Next he can ask each of the partners, "Whereabouts on the island would you like to spend time if your relationship was in a better place?" Each of the partners indicates a preferred location, and the therapist marks them with playing pieces. "In order to achieve that, you'd need to move from here to there." The therapist points from the places on the island where the clients have spent a lot of their time up until now over to the places where they'd like to go. He can ask, "What do you think, should your husband go and fetch you from where you have previously been, or will you come and meet him? Will you meet each other in the middle, in between your previous locations, or somewhat further away, heading towards your destination? Would it be easier if your wife came to meet you or if she allowed you to travel over to where she's been spending most of her time so far?" The therapist keeps the couple's attention on the map during this process, which tends to avoid any discussion of "real life". The therapist can then continue: "You're heading to different destinations ... will you go to your wife's destination together first and then to yours, or vice versa? Will you go there sometimes alone and sometimes as a couple, or will you go everywhere together? Will you arrange to meet up between your destination and your husband's destination, or sometimes in one place and sometimes in the other? Will you first go to his location and then stay longer in yours, or the other way round, or a completely different arrangement?"

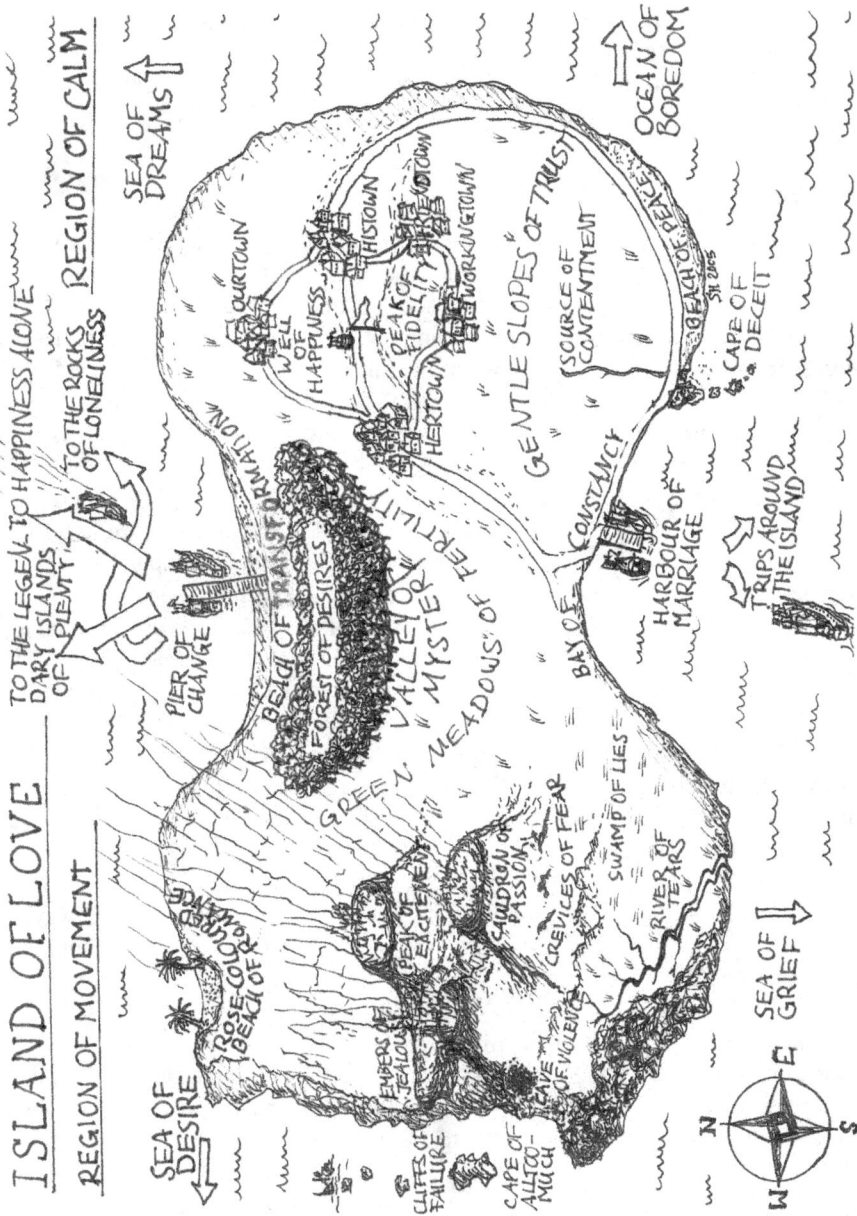

Figure 8.5 The Island of Love

It is rare for a couple to return to their previous style of discussion following a conversation of this kind. Instead, what tends to happen in my experience is that after a while the partners – even when talking about "real life" – discuss solutions and resources and express confidence and the desire for mutual support.

If an intervention of this kind[23] is carried out during a video call, the therapist can make available a photo or PowerPoint presentation of the map using the screen-share function or direct his camera at a map or flipchart in his room.

8.3.2 Self-produced island maps

It goes without saying that island maps of this kind can also be self-produced by couples or individuals. It is a good idea to ask clients, "If you were to visualise your situation as an island map, which landscape elements would belong on it?" If the therapist starts by giving a couple of examples, it's likely that the list will grow rapidly; there might be some "meadows of happiness", for example, or some "fog patches of ignorance", a "lighthouse of wisdom" or a "swamp of ambiguity".

The therapist can start by drawing up a list of a few dozen landscape labels of this kind together with the client.

Then the therapist or the client can sketch the outlines of the island before annotating it with the landscape elements, using simple symbols that are labelled accordingly. The client decides where these places are located. If she is extremely indecisive (as is to be expected in the context of stresses relating to depression, for example), the therapist can propose and draw in locations, distinguishing in the process between a "peninsula of change (movement)" and a "peninsula of permanence (calm)".

Now the therapist can work together with the client to think about which changes are necessary; what is needed in terms of transport links, telephone lines, shipping services for outside contact, a renaturing programme, a tourism project …?

How would the island map change if these measures were put into practice? The therapist or the client can mark the appropriate symbols and labels on the map.

The therapist can ask,

"How will the life of the people living there alter if the island changes in this way? What effect will that have on their relationships, on their self-confidence, and on their behaviour?"

This brings us to the following systemic questions.

What will change for the client if she looks at her life through the lens of this metaphor and with this physiology? Assuming that what she experiences and how she behaves over the next few weeks fits this attitude to life, what will change?

The guano islands (child therapy)

A seven-year-old boy came to therapy because he often soiled himself. According to his mother, whenever it happened he would claim somewhat flippantly that it had just happened, and he didn't know why. The boy seemed embarrassed to me, and the subject was visibly an unpleasant one for him. I told the boy and his mother about the "guano islands", which for many millions of years have been a resting place for seagulls after a hard day's fishing. I asked whether he could imagine what it looked like there. The islands were covered in heaps of seagull poop measuring many metres in height. A resourceful businessman discovered that this poop was the best fertiliser in the world. So he transported excavators there to remove the guano and tip it onto trucks. From there it goes into freight containers, and a crane lifts the containers onto a ship. When the ship is full, it takes the poop to people in Europe, who pay a lot of money for it. In the port of these guano islands there's a clock so that the excavator operators know how much time they have to fill a truck before the next one comes along, and so that the truck drivers know how much time they have to bring the poop to the container, and so that the captains know when they need to make space for the next ship that arrives. Once the whole island is free of poop, they're able to take the excavators and trucks to the next island and repeat the whole process there. The aim is to build a park on the well-fertilised island and to construct houses where people can live. In order to ensure that this all happens, they use helicopters to chase away the seagulls so that they poop where it doesn't bother people, and not where people want to live. I asked the mother to sit down together with the boy and draw a map of the island showing how far the excavators had already progressed with their work. In the event of a relapse, they should talk about what was currently happening on the island. Most importantly, however, they should regularly update the map with the progress made over the next few weeks and months …[24]

The Daniel island (adolescent therapy)

"If your life were an island, what would you need to draw on a map of the island?" I asked Daniel, a teenager who had been diagnosed with autism.

"Anger. Hatred. Devastation."

"And fear? Loneliness?"
  "Maybe."
  "Anything else?"
  "School-related stuff. Annoying teachers. Revision for A-Levels."
We carried on like that for a while.

"So perhaps we could draw a volcano on the island, with three craters: the 'Anger Crater', the 'Hatred Crater' and the 'Devastation Crater'. Is that OK?"
"Yep."

First I drew in the volcanoes, before adding additional landscape elements.

"And next to that maybe the 'Crevices of Fear' and the 'Grotto of Loneliness'?"
"Yeah, that too."

"The 'School Desert'?"

"It's more like a lunar landscape."

"OK, so the 'Lunar Landscape of School-Related Stuff'."

"Yeah."

"Is there a teacher's village there, or do the teachers have their own island?"

"Their own island would be better."

"OK then, the 'Island of Teachers'. Then we'd also need an 'Island of Pupils' for the other pupils. And an 'Island of Parents'?"

"Yeah, probably."

"An 'Island of Other People'?"

"Sure."

"Sometimes we need to come into contact with others, after all. What else might it be good to have there? A harbour with ferry connections to the other islands? A submarine harbour? A bridge? A helipad?"

"Probably all of them would be a good idea. A bridge might be a bit tricky though …"

"So a harbour for ships, a harbour for submarines and a helipad. One of each on each island. What about roads? I'm sure you'd need some of them on your island to connect up the different bits."

"We could have one going from right to left and one from top to bottom, and a crossroads in the middle."

"And a house where someone can live at the crossroads? Or one at the ends of each of the roads?"

"Both, one in the centre and one at each end. Then you'd have a choice …"

"What would you do for a phone connection? Mobile or landline?"

"A mobile connection would be more practical."

"Yes, then you'd also be able to call the other islands. So we'd need a phone mast on your island and one on every other island …"[25]

The family island (family therapy)

The therapist can draw a "family island" together with those present at a family therapy session. He should start by taking a large sheet of paper and drawing the outlines of such an island, and then ask for the names of prominent locations. Either he can draw in the locations himself after consulting everyone present, or the family member who suggested the locations can do so.

If a family member reacts in a disparaging manner to the name of a location that has been suggested, the suggestion can be adapted by finding a terminology that everyone can agree on (reframing). In order to do so, it can be helpful to identify the good intention or the need (self-preservation, belonging) behind an undesirable behaviour.

The therapist can ask the family members to guess where the others would be located at a particular point in time (currently, during a conflict, mostly).

"What do you think your father would say if I asked him where he was at this time?" (circular questioning). He could then put the question to the relevant individual.

The family members can be asked individually where they would like to spend more or less time, when they would like to travel together and when separately, and how they could greet each other or step aside in a friendly fashion. The points that have been discussed can be visualised by drawing in roads, tunnels, telephone lines, and other infrastructure elements. If the island map has been placed on the floor or on a table, the positions of the family members can be marked using playing figures in various different colours. If a flipchart has been used, the same can be done with Post-it notes.

Experiences of violence or other stressful events can be described as volcanic eruptions, storms, catastrophic floods, or earthquakes. The resulting damage can be marked in on the map and described. As in the case of the "mountain village" intervention outlined below, a discussion can be held on the clean-up and renovation tasks that are necessary, and how the tasks should be divided up between the clean-up workers so that the outcome is successful. It is a good idea always to remain "in character" (i.e. using the terminology of the metaphor) so that solutions can be found spontaneously without taking a circuitous route involving accusations and justifications.

A further option is to consider what might be necessary or desirable to develop the island (economically, for tourists, with a view to quality of life).

8.3.3 The mountain village

I use the story about the renovation of a mountain village damaged by a mudflow *inter alia* with clients suffering from symptoms of depression, trauma-related anxiety, and sudden severe illnesses, as well as in relationship counselling, in order to help clients find a new way of dealing with stressful memories, grief phenomena, self-reproaches, distrust, anger, the effort of self-regeneration, and the fear of a recurring disaster.

"Imagine a village high up in the mountains, alongside a stream and among green meadows, surrounded by snow-capped peaks. Sometimes it suffers from a problem known by those who live in the Alps as a mudflow; while the snow is melting or if it rains a lot, a stream like this can turn into a rushing torrent carrying with it mud, stones, rocks and tree trunks, which can cause immense damage to a village. The residents can save themselves since they know what is coming, which gives them a few hours to gather together their most treasured possessions and get themselves to safety, but the village is severely affected. Once the water levels have fallen, the village residents take a look at the damage. Then they assemble and discuss what should be done. I imagine that would look something like this …" (Figure 8.6).

Time axis/film/from now on:	Spatial axis/river/up until now:
Transformation of the village	Back story of the village –
• from damaged to healed,	a catastrophe that came with a warning. Now:
• from at risk to safe,	flood protection as healing of expectation,
• from unhappy to happy	erosion protection as healing of
	• film memory
	• bodily memories (learned reflexes, trigger reactions)

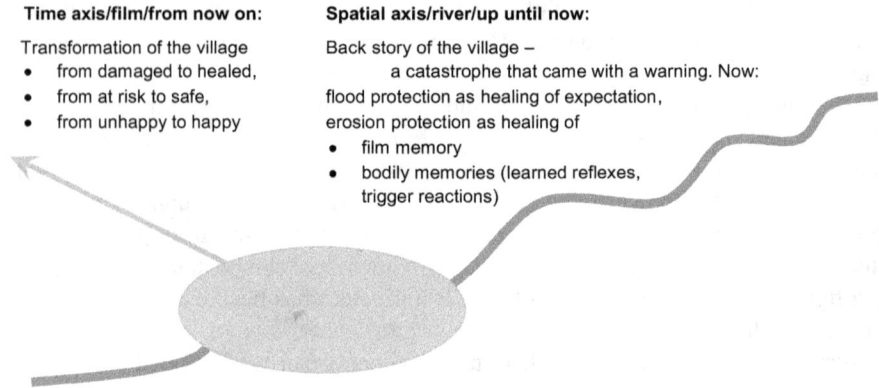

Figure 8.6 The mountain village

The structure of this renovation story can be outlined as follows.

0. Disaster

a) Getting to safety
b) Returning
c) Inspecting the damage

1. Clearing away the rubble

a) Using excavators, trucks, wheelbarrows, shovels, cranes
b) Using hoses, pressure washers
c) Visit by the structural engineer

2. Tradespeople

a) Bricklayers, carpenters, roofers, window fitters
b) Electricians, plumbers
c) Drain cleaners, road builders, bridge builders
d) Painters, landscape gardeners
e) Anything else?

3. Commemoration

a) High-water mark, bronze plaque, rock, sculpture, fountain, tree?
b) Village square, side road, cemetery, at the stream, in the museum, outdoors?
c) Dedication with the parish priest, mayor, Alpine horn players?
d) Laying of a wreath on the anniversary? Opportunity for anyone who feels the need to light a candle?
e) None of the above?
f) Two memorials? (Sometimes useful in relationship counselling or family therapy)

4. Prevention

a) Make the stream deeper and wider?

b) Flood wall, sandbags?

c) Flood zone on the meadows above the village? Dam?

d) Bypass channel? Underground, under the meadow, through a tunnel to another valley?

e) Shrubs along the stream right the way to the source as protection against erosion? Or steel mesh?

f) Divers who search for loose material in the caves at the source of the stream? Measures to restrain the material? Blasting?

5. Village festival

a) Schuhplattler dancers, yodelling group? More modern music? Dancing?

b) Performances by clubs, school classes, drama groups?

c) Coffee, cakes? Free beer?

d) Lanterns, decorations?

e) Anything else?

8.3.4 Idiomatic landscapes

Proverbs and sayings are a rich source of problem landscape metaphors.

Clients often introduce landscapes of this kind into the discussion unconsciously, as follows.

"I'm drowning in work …"

"My husband has shut himself up in his ivory tower."

"I've been left high and dry."

Most of these idioms describe scenes where a person is at the mercy of a situation in which he suffers harm. They sketch out the elements of the landscape in which this suffering takes place. The images that are conjured up when such idioms are used have a direct effect on the client's dream world, which is where they originated. Metaphors of powerlessness, together with the landscape into which they are incorporated, can be transformed into metaphors of creativity.

Situations and landscapes that are described idiomatically can be reshaped in three different ways: following a rules-based logic, an exception-based logic, and a cartoon-based logic.

Reframing in keeping with a rules-based logic involves paying attention to circumstances that alter the situation and the landscape based on certain rules.

An exception-based logic means that we describe how things might happen exceptionally in an unusual way.

A cartoon-based logic means that we outline how something might happen in our imagination, without worrying too much about the rules of everyday logic.

If the client says, "I've been left high and dry," and we respond, "If we take that metaphor very literally for once, what can you see in front of your inner eye?", she might say, "I'm sitting on a hill in a desert."

Following a *rules-based logic*, we can answer, "There's an area of desert in the Middle East where irrigation systems have been installed that can be used to extend the arable zone ever further into the desert. A very similar thing is happening with the afforestation programme at the edge of the Sahel. Now imagine yourself drilling wells, laying pipes and hoses, hanging up nets to provide shade, working the land and irrigating it. How will the landscape change?"

Following an *exception-based logic*, we can say, "In the Arabian Desert they once bored down to a depth of a thousand metres to find oil. They didn't find any oil, but instead they hit a geyser of water. So they built an oasis with surrounding parkland and adjacent agricultural areas. If you imagine this borehole in your dry zone, what do you see?"

Following a *cartoon-based logic*, we can say, "Now we both know you're not really sitting in the desert – you're sitting here in this room with a window, a floor, and a chair. Strictly speaking, it's not you that's in the desert, but instead the desert is a cartoon in your head. Please ask your internal director to take over the task of transforming the desert into a beautiful landscape that benefits you. What can you see there?"[26]

The outcomes of interventions like this are often extremely impressive; the metaphors now have a liberating rather than a paralysing effect. The client's entire physiology alters. Her emotions and bodily reactions seem to have been replaced, so that they now fit the new metaphor and run counter to those that were associated with the initial metaphor. This effect persists even if the client is asked again about the initial topic (the "problem"), provided that the new experience is prioritised over the problem memory when the question is asked. The therapist can ask the following questions (while sounding curious, happy, hopeful, and expectant).

"If you think about your initial situation now, with this metaphor in mind, how do you feel?"

"If you'd already had that attitude to life when you arrived at our session today, what would your problem be now? Supposing that were the case, what's next for you?"

"If you arrive at the exam as the person who you are in this landscape, what's changed?"

"If we ask your brain to connect this experience with a feeling that things have always been like that and they obviously couldn't be any different, what else do you need?"

Visiting idiomatic landscapes

At the start of this section, we discussed a number of idioms that clients use to describe their problems (such as "being left high and dry"). The therapist can proceed as follows to ensure that these sayings can be put to therapeutic use.

He can suggest to himself that he should turn on his "ear for metaphors", which alerts him every time that an idiom is used, or his "internal photographer", who takes stills of the resulting daydream. What does he think the problem landscape might look like?

- If the client talks about "being left high and dry", "dried out inside", or "sent into the wilderness", it might be a desert.
- If she talks about a "sinking ship", "shipwreck", "going down with the ship", or "being up to his neck in it", it might be a sea or another body of water.
- If she talks about a "gilded cage", "being trapped", or "being sentenced", it might be a prison or something similar.
- If she talks about "being ruined", a "wreck", or a "construction site", it might be a building undergoing renovation. Based on this, what does the solution landscape look like?

If the problem landscape is ...

- a *desert*, the solution landscape is an *oasis*.
- a *sea*, the solution landscape is an *island*.[27]
- a *prison*, then the solution landscape is the *world of freedom* outside the prison gates.
- a *building undergoing renovation*, then the solution landscape is the *renovated building*.

Assuming that the client succeeds in finding a route out of the problem landscape and into the solution landscape, what will happen to lead her there?

What will be the first step towards salvation, what will be the second, and how will it continue?

The client can be guided by the therapist into the solution zone in a narrative style (monologue) or in a conversational style (dialogue).

The journey to the solution landscape (narrative style)

If the therapist chooses a narrative style, it is a good idea to use a story with a happy ending in keeping with a rules-based or exception-based logic. If the client says that her ship ran aground, the therapist – following a rules-based logic – can recount how certain seafarers were rescued and what stories they later told about the accident involving their ship. In keeping with an exception-based logic, he can also talk about how the history of seafaring features repeated instances of dolphins rescuing people in distress at sea, and make conjectures about how they manage to pull off these rescues.

Other idioms can similarly be used as a starting point, for example by talking about someone who found his way out of a desert, escaped from prison, or repaired a building that was falling down, either in line with the rules of survival or by a stroke of luck.

It is a relatively straightforward task to plot the route from the problem landscape to the solution landscape if the aforementioned six steps are kept in mind. As a reminder:

1. Introduce the *protagonist* and his world!
2. Refer to the protagonist's *problem*!
3. Describe the unsuccessful *attempts to find a solution*!
4. Make clear the protagonist's *misfortune*!
5. Present an internal or external helper with a new *resource*!
6. Reveal a *success* – or leave the outcome open for further thought!

The journey to the solution landscape (dialogue style)

If the therapist decides to carry out the intervention in the form of a dialogue, he will ask the client questions. He can ask a client who says that her ship has "run aground", "If you imagine taking that metaphor very literally, what do you see?" The subsequent questions are formulated in such a way that all of the anticipated answers bring the client closer to a happy ending for her internal film. For example, the therapist will probably not ask, "Now that you've left the sinking ship, can you still swim, or are you already close to drowning?", but instead, "In the event of a maritime disaster, there's normally a heap of junk floating around: cargo, furniture, parts of the ship, life belts, lifeboats … What might be a good thing to grab and hold tight to?" "Seafarers are often rescued by other boats, but sometimes also by helicopters and sometimes by swimming to shore. Which of these do you think might be true for you?"

The therapist can carry on developing the story with the client like this until the client can celebrate her rescue. He should always phrase his questions with the following in mind: assuming that the story has a happy ending, what needs to happen next?

Transforming idiomatic landscapes (documentary film technique)

If it appears permissible to change perspective in this manner, the therapist can also ask, "Are you familiar with the ship named the *Vasa*? They finished building it in 1628, and it was one of the largest and most heavily armed warships of its time. It was launched in Stockholm, set sail – and sank after only twenty minutes. That was no joke at the time. Many years later, however, it became possible to salvage the wreck and restore it. Today it's housed in a museum built specially for the purpose. Its previous splendour has been newly restored."

This allows the therapist – without needing to verbalise it – to initiate an internal search in the client aimed at discovering how whatever is currently being experienced as a disaster might later be beneficial in some way or at least be admired with interest.[28]

Transforming idiomatic landscapes (cartoon technique)

The therapist might also say to a client, "Strictly speaking, of course, you're not in the sea (can you see any waves here?), but instead the sea with you in it is inside you, like a cartoon in your head. If we asked your internal director to try and adapt the film so that it benefits you, what would she need to do? I know it might sound crazy, but let's try imagining it. Should she arrange for a big plug to be pulled out so that all the water runs out as though it were draining out of a bathtub, so that you can then walk back to civilisation by foot? Or would it be better for her to hire an eagle that will grab your belt and carry you to the nearest island?"

Transforming idiomatic landscapes (superposition technique)

The idioms used by the client are useful starting points in this connection. They are not a vital prerequisite for techniques of this kind, however. Instead, the therapist can simply ask a question similar to the following:

"If the way you're feeling now were a landscape, how would it look?" "What else can you see there?" "Anything else?"

The client will then describe a problem landscape. The therapist can continue with the following questions:

"If your internal director who showed you this landscape could make a different landscape out of it that would be beneficial to you, what would it look like?" "What else can you see there?" "Anything else?" "And can you hear anything …?" "If you take a look around in this landscape, what is it like?" "How does that feel now?"

The client now describes the solution landscape, with her mood visibly improving as she does so. Finally, the therapist can ask the following questions:

"Would it be OK if you asked your brain to hold onto this feeling, and possibly even to strengthen it a bit more? Do you think your brain is OK with that?"[29]

8.4 Therapeutic spaces

"The more perceptible the therapy, the more effective it is."[30] In keeping with this rule, it is a good idea to use not only imagined or drawn spaces, but also the therapy room. Ropes and symbols (or markings without any contextual significance) can be used to structure the room, or three-dimensional models can be generated from objects that exemplify problem experiences and potential solutions.

The entire room should be used for the following line models, spatial area models, and circle models. Anything that is experienced in a setting of this kind is perceived as relating to the whole of a client's existence or life or the entire world. It follows that interventions of this kind are very powerful, but can, however, also be risky if the therapist does not act cautiously. As a precaution, in the event that the client re-experiences traumatic memories as a result of age regression, it is a good idea to agree neutral zones by stating that anyone standing in a particular location is "out of the game".

8.4.1 Line models

One option for structuring the room is to visualise chronologies spatially. When doing so, a rope can be used as an axis along which the consecutive events are depicted ("lifeline"), or the quantitative component of time can be ignored and its experiential quality emphasised ("river of life").

Lifeline

The following procedure is based on timeline models that are popular in coaching and management training sessions, but has been modified for hypnosystemic purposes.[31]

1. The therapist discusses the client's current situation and objective with her.
2. The therapist or the client places a rope in the room that represents the client's lifeline. The therapist asks the client which points of the rope should represent the past, the future, and the present moment, and then asks her to choose a symbol to mark the current moment.
3. Keeping in mind the objective of the therapy, the therapist asks the client to mark important memories from her past life on one side of the rope. If the client mentions stressful experiences, these are marked on the other side of the rope. The client's conception and birth can be marked at the start of the rope.
4. The therapist asks the client to mark a point in the future at which she has achieved her objective (in her imagination), and another showing an objective behind the objective. A time of death is not marked because it is not known or planned, and should not be suggested (unless the client wants to take a grateful look back on her fulfilled life from her death bed).
5. The client walks along the rope ("chronologically") on the resources side, and comments on the connection between the marked situations and her goal. Once she has arrived in the present, the therapist asks her to look back at the past. Character-building and stressful experiences can be contemplated with pride and thankfulness for what has been achieved and overcome.
6. The therapist invites the client to stand in the present and look forwards into a good future where her objective is achieved or her problem is solved.
7. He asks her to stand at the objective and to look back at the present and the past, and then to stand at the objective behind the objective and look back, and in each case to describe her impressions.
8. The therapist asks the client to position herself at locations along the rope that feel strong and good, to soak up this experience into herself and to transport it to the locations where it is needed, regardless of whether good is taken from the past to the future, from the future to the past, from the past or future to the present, from earlier futures or pasts to later futures or pasts or vice versa.
9. The therapist asks the client to stand in the location where she would like to end the work, to soak up everything she has experienced that is good and to take it with her to use during the rest of her life.

River of life

The following procedure is based on the river of life model by Peter Nemetschek. It is designed in particular for couples and families, but also for individuals who wish to work on their relationships with family members or other people.[32]

1. The therapist talks to the clients about their biographical situation and objectives.
2. He places a rope in the room for the oldest person as a lifeline (or two ropes for the family's parents). The therapist is responsible for handling of the ropes so that he can respectfully reframe any self-depreciation or mutual criticism, and shape an interpretation of the situation that is mutually agreeable to all parties involved.
3. He places ropes for the other parties involved alongside, with a staggered starting position to indicate their later birth dates. The precise course that should be followed by the rope is then discussed; ought the rope to bend a little to the right or to the left at this point? Where might a meander express a crisis (e.g. at the present location, since it was a crisis that brought the family to therapy)? Where does the river tend to follow a straighter course?
4. The therapist explains that the ropes visualise the river of life from its source to the sea, and that rivers have meanders. The meandering of the ropes can represent the proximity and distance of the individuals to each other over the course of their lives. When do they flow away from each other, and when are they very close? During periods of separation (or before a couple had met, for example), the ropes are far apart. The rope representing a child who is sometimes closer to her mother and sometimes to her father can move back and forth between their ropes. If a child has broken off contact with a parent, this can be expressed by moving the child's rope to the other side of the other parent's rope. Distant and unknown parents are placed some way away. Relationships that are not to be strengthened (damaging extra-marital affairs) are marked with symbols, and ropes are not laid down for them.
5. While talking to the clients, the therapist shapes a biography from the perspective of proximity and distance, and reframes everything derogatory in a respectful manner. He asks each of the clients to select symbols (e.g. semi-precious stones) as markers, and to place these at the locations they have chosen.
6. He invites the clients to consider the following questions: where are you now? Still in the middle of the current meander of the river, or perhaps just beyond it? Over the course of the discussion, a location is jointly identified where the present should be marked with a symbol.

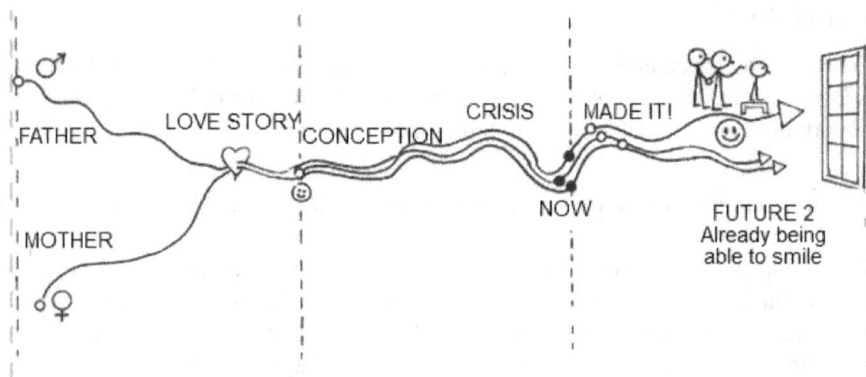

Figure 8.7 The river of life

7. The future is located according to the aspirations of those involved. If these latter are not consistent, an option that is acceptable to everyone is used instead, with a reminder that it is not intended to dictate any particular route. (If it proves difficult to reach an agreement, forking paths can also be added to represent potential routes that individuals could decide to take.)
8. The therapist asks the partners to jointly ("synchronously") position themselves at locations or times in the past, present, and future that they assume might feel helpful for everyone involved, to look at each other and to look together into the past and future while standing there, and to talk about their experiences of the various perspectives.
9. The therapist can also invite the clients to fill themselves up with the good from one period and transport it to locations in another period. Clients can move together or follow different routes when doing so, provided that anything regarded by one of them as a resource is viewed favourably by the other.
10. Clients are asked to go and stand where they would like to end the work, to soak up all the good that they have experienced and to take it with them to use during the rest of their lives.

Other options include the addition of ramps and waterfalls, loops and spirals (Figure 8.7).

Knots often tend to have negative implications. Clients can experience their positive future by standing on a raised stool or platform. They can take with them a symbol of success or luck as an anchor, such as a precious stone.

8.4.2 Spatial area models

Another option is to divide the room up into different areas, and then to assign different meanings to these areas.

The corridor

I often use the following intervention for clients with concerns or diagnoses associated with having too low or too high a level of demand or structure in their lives, *inter alia*:

- Asperger's/autism,
- ADD and ADHD,
- dyslexia and dyscalculia,
- being highly gifted and highly sensitive,
- hyperacusis and other forms of sensitivity to stimuli,
- boredom and work stress, boreout and burnout,
- perfectionism and obsessiveness.

1. The therapist places a rope on the floor in the centre of the room. He explains that the rope marks the boundary between the spheres of life where the level of demand is too high and those where it is too low.
2. The therapist asks the client to stand on the side that she perceives as less of a "problem", and asks her to describe how she feels there. He also mirrors back to the client any bodily reactions he notices in her during this process.
3. He invites the client to move over to the side that she perceives as more of a "problem", and again to describe how she feels there. If necessary, he can repeat the process of mirroring back to her anything he spots in terms of her bodily reactions while she is in this location.
4. He places a second rope parallel to the first, and explains that this area is a corridor between low demand and high demand (or between low structure and high structure). He asks the client to step in and describe what it feels like there.
5. If necessary, he can ask the client to place one leg in the area of low demand and one in the central zone, and to describe the difference between the two halves of the body. Then he can repeat the procedure with the area of high demand and the central zone.
6. The therapist places the ropes further apart. He asks the client to walk around between them and to verbalise anything that has changed. Then he places the ropes directly against the walls, asks the client to walk around between them again and to describe her experience.
7. If necessary, he can suggest to the client that the ropes might be taken away, since the room in any case now consists only of the central zone. He asks the client to experience what it feels like now to wander around in the room. He talks to her about how she can take this experience everywhere with her. If necessary, he can walk with the client into other rooms or to her car, and ask her to confirm that the good experience is still there wherever she goes.

The four quadrants

The following intervention is a little more elaborate. It is nevertheless well worth the effort of becoming familiar with it and trying it out, since it has proven exceptionally beneficial in therapeutic terms. I use it in particular for people who come to me with the following:

- addiction issues,
- eating disorders,
- obsessiveness and perfectionist tendencies,
- burnout and work–life balance issues,
- a desire to find a life where the level of demand placed upon them is neither too high nor too low (see above), procrastination.

1. The therapist places a rope on the ground that divides the room into a structured area (e.g. successful) and an unstructured area (e.g. addicted).
2. He asks the client to position herself on one side of the rope, and to describe how she feels there. The therapist can add his own observations about the client's bodily reactions.
3. He then asks the client to position herself on the other side of the rope and to describe how she feels there. Once again, he can add anything he notices in terms of bodily reactions.
4. The therapist then places a second rope on the floor, crosswise to the first. He explains that this marks the boundary between the advantages and disadvantages of the two sides.

This results in four quadrants:

A: Advantages of the structured area, e.g. experience of success, recognition, realisation of certain values	B: Disadvantages of the structured area, e.g. exhaustion, loneliness, disappointment about lack of recognition and the fact that values are not shared by others
C: Advantages of the unstructured area, e.g. enjoyment, comfort, celebration, relaxation, experience of freedom	D: Disadvantages of the unstructured area, e.g. shame, loss of control, health and relationship problems

5. The therapist asks the client to step into Quadrants A, B, C, and D one after another, and then into Quadrant A again (in this order, or in other words tracing out a figure of eight), and to notice and describe the bodily sensations and attitudes to life that fit with each quadrant.
6. While the client steps between the quadrants for a second time, the therapist can provide an explanation similar to the following:

"If we were to describe what you are experiencing in a model, it might go something like this.

A: You experience success and recognition in what you are doing, and because that feels good, you do more of it, until … (move to Quadrant B!)

B: ... you're exhausted, disappointed, and frustrated because of the difficulties associated with that ... (now move to Quadrant C!)

C: ... and so you want to console yourself and relax in the evening and celebrate what you have achieved, and because that feels good, you do more of it, until ... (now move to Quadrant D!)

D: ... you get into a state you're ashamed of or feel guilty about, or which is not good for you in some other way, and in order to compensate for that ... (now move to Quadrant A!)

A: ... on the following day you demonstrate what you're capable of doing, which makes you feel like you are in fact valuable, until it all becomes too much and you go back to Quadrant B again ...

Is that making any sense to you?"

7. The therapist asks the client to fill herself up to the top with the good experience in Quadrant A, to transport it over to Quadrant D by stepping diagonally across, to spread it out there and to feel what changes. He asks the client to describe the change.

The therapist can explain (in words to this effect): "You have everything you need for a happy life. The only problem so far has been that it's not been where you've needed it. We've moved the resources from Zone A to Zone D, which means that your skills – prioritisation, setting boundaries, planning, imposing structure and control – are where they're needed. This means that you no longer need to get to the point where shame and guilt come into play, and so you no longer need to compensate on the following day until disappointment and exhaustion appear."

A: **Advantages of the structured area, e.g. experience of success, recognition, realisation of certain values**	B: Disadvantages of the structured area, e.g. exhaustion, loneliness, disappointment about lack of recognition and the fact that values are not shared by others
C: Advantages of unstructured area, e.g. enjoyment, comfort, celebration, relaxation, experience of freedom	D: **Disadvantages of the unstructured area, e.g. shame, loss of control, health and relationship problems**

8. Now the therapist asks the client to fill herself up to the top with the good experience in Quadrant C, to transport it over to Quadrant B by stepping diagonally across, to spread it out there and to feel what changes. He asks the client to describe the change.

The therapist can explain (in words to this effect): "We've taken the resources from Zone C, or in other words the capacity to feel encouragement, joy, pleasure, and relaxation, to Zone B, where there was previously exhaustion and disappointment.

Since your brain organises it in such a way that you have the pleasant experiences even while you are at work, you no longer need to compensate by catching up on them at the end of the working day. That also means that you no longer reach the point of shame and guilty feelings ..."

A: Advantages of the structured area, e.g. experience of success, recognition, realisation of certain values	B: **Disadvantages of the structured area, e.g. exhaustion, loneliness, disappointment about lack of recognition and the fact that values are not shared by others**
C: **Advantages of unstructured area, e.g. enjoyment, comfort, celebration, relaxation, experience of freedom**	D: Disadvantages of the unstructured area, e.g. shame, loss of control, health and relationship problems

9. The therapist asks the client to place one foot in one quadrant (e.g. Quadrant A) and the other foot in another quadrant (e.g. Quadrant B), and to decide whether the two halves of the body feel the same or different. If one half of the body feels better than the other, the client should make the experience from the more pleasant quadrant rise up to her head and then send it to the other side of her body, right down to her fingers and toes, and then on into the surrounding quadrant, until the two halves of the body feel the same.

If Quadrants A and C are being compared, the advantages of each side can be taken across to the other side in a combined movement; similarly, if Quadrants B and D are being compared, the advantages associated with the absence of the other side's disadvantages can be taken across.

10. The client can again wander around between the quadrants, and take away the ropes if all the quadrants feel equally good. The therapist can ask what is different now compared to the start of the session, and share any observations of his own.

8.4.3 Circle models

Another option for structuring the room is to distinguish between different opportunities for action or different possible experiences by visualising them as circles in the room. This can be achieved in the form of a "problem circle and resource circle" (where stressful and strengthening memories are differentiated from each other) or in the form of a "tetralemma" (where different options for action are differentiated from each other).

Problem circle and resource circle (force surge)

It is recommended that the steps of this intervention should be sequenced in such a way that the resources are dealt with at the start.[33] The client can be reminded that she can also step outside both of the circles at any time in order to return to a neutral experience. This ensures that the procedure is structured in a gentle and safe fashion, with due regard for any traumas suffered by the client. The procedure takes the following form.

1. The therapist asks the client to name a problem experience as well as a particularly good resource (a success, a happy memory, a loved person).
2. He asks her to use pieces of rope or wool to place two circles on the ground next to each other. The circles designate the resource experience and the problem experience.
3. He asks her to step into the resource experience circle and to describe what is associated with this experience, in particular her bodily sensations and her emotions.
4. Then he asks her to step out of that circle. Before testing out the problem circle, the therapist emphasises that the client's internal self will regulate the experience in such a way that nothing will ever get too much, and that she can return to the zone outside the circle whenever she wants. The therapist asks the client to step into the problem circle and to describe what she experiences here, in particular her bodily sensations and her emotions. This step can be omitted if the experience was particularly traumatic or the client voices serious misgivings about stepping into the circle.
5. The therapist asks the client to step into the resource circle again, to fill herself up right to the top with the experience felt there, and then to take a big step and transport it over to the problem circle and spread it out there. He asks her to describe what changes in terms of her bodily sensations, her emotions, and her perception of her surroundings.

The intervention can also be designed to feature several resource circles and one problem circle. In this case the client would step from one resource circle to the next and "gather" the resources from the different circles into her body before moving over to the problem circle. The client can repeatedly bring helpful experiences from the resource circle over to the problem circle one after another or, in order to speed up the process and once the first resources have been brought over, pull more and more positive energy over into the problem circle using an invisible conduit.

The tetralemma

Tetralemma work originated with Matthias Varga von Kibéd and Insa Sparrer.[34] It is particularly appropriate for people who regard themselves as indecisive or ambivalent towards a possible decision (which is potentially experienced as necessary). One variation of this tetralemma work takes the following form.

1. The therapist asks the client to mark locations on the ground for the following options, using ropes or symbols:

- "The One"
- "The Other"

- "As well – As" ("All / Both")
- "None of them" ("Neither" / "Neither – Nor")
- "None of these, and that neither"

2. The therapist asks the client to stand in all the different locations one after another, to sense with her body how they feel, and to perceive what changes when moving from each of the locations to the others.
3. For example, he can ask which associations occur to the client in each location, which impulses she feels, which internal voices she hears, and which emotions are fitting in each case.
4. He also asks the client to walk through the areas between the markings. He invites her to find the best position – on a marking, between the markings, half on and half in between two markings etc. ... He then asks the client to describe her experiences and associations again. The client stands in the best location that has been found, and the good there is felt and intensified. She is asked to intensify it only as much as she wants, and then to step over into the "real" world of the present moment with this good feeling.

Alternatively, the client can place rope circles that are experienced positively around each other or overlapping each other, after which she should find the best arrangement for herself under such conditions.

The five positions would then be as shown in Figure 8.8.

8.4.4 Three-dimensional spatial models

Most three-dimensional spatial models do not use the entire room, but instead present a concrete model offering a new perspective on the problem and its solutions, or open up fresh possibilities for solving the problem.

Six rods

If a client believes that she has no options (for example, that she cannot quit her job because she is too old), the therapist can give her six rods of equal length, and ask her to arrange them in four triangles. If the client gets stuck, the therapist can give her the following clue: "Would it help if I gave you a bit of plasticine as well?" The problem can be solved by making a three-sided pyramid.

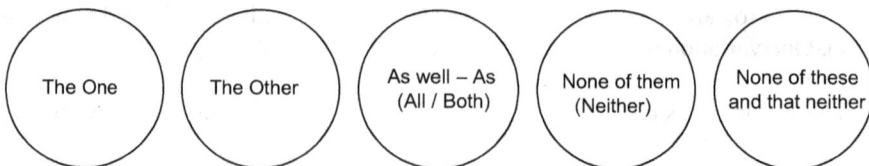

Figure 8.8 Tetralemma

The plasticine is used to stabilise the sculpture. This sculpture will then be present during the remainder of the therapy session as a silent and vivid reminder of the fact that even problems that appear insoluble can in fact be solved.

At equilibrium

Sometimes couples come to therapy and want to know whether their relationship has any future. They express concerns because the woman is older than the man or the man is much older than the woman, because they come from two different cultural backgrounds or because they live a long way away from each other. It is difficult to predict whether such relationships might go the distance. It should merely be remembered that any prediction made by the therapist will have a certain tendency to become self-fulfilling. Instead of spending lots of time talking about it, the therapist can instead slot a spoon, a fork (or two forks), and a match inside one another and balance the whole contraption on the edge of a wine glass, allow the couple a moment or two to observe the miracle, and then say, "Some things work even if you have no idea why they work."[35]

It's a good idea to practice this trick once or twice before performing it to clients. It goes without saying that a model of this kind can be applied in many different situations, for example if a client mentions that she must regain her balance, find her equilibrium, or achieve a balance between the different parts of her life, or that only a miracle can help her, she's facing an impossible task and so on.

8.5 Therapeutic modelling

During therapeutic modelling …

- stresses are personified, taken out of the body and described (subtraction procedure),
- dissociated stresses are divided up (subtraction outside the client),
- resources are personified and placed in the room, described, perceived as an experience of identity, and stabilised (addition procedure),
- personified stresses outside the client are transformed into resources (transformation procedure).

In order to identify what changes as a result of the relevant intervention, bodily reactions are observed, and the client is asked about any alterations in her experience that are perceived as useful or less useful.

If the work is being carried out during a video or phone call, the client should position the imagined persons in her own room. It is enough for the therapist to know which individual persons are there – he does not need to know exactly where they are. When working with couples, families, or teams, it is a good idea to agree on the location where each imagined person is standing, so that the different partners or different members of the family or team have the same point of reference when it comes to trying out different locations. Work of this kind is easier if they are sitting together in front of a *single* screen. If they are in different locations, the following agreement can be reached: "Let's imagine that you're sitting together on a sofa, with Mrs X on the right and Mr X on the left ..."[36]

8.5.1 Subtraction of symptoms

The most common application of the subtraction procedure is to dissociate symptoms described in physical, mental, or social terms from the client, to ask her to experience how she feels without them, and to stabilise this experience or to develop it further in a helpful manner during the remainder of the conversation.

Asking the exhausted one to sit over there

The following procedure is based on the therapeutic modelling procedure of subtraction (dissociation in keeping with the principle of "separating problems").

A 23-year-old woman from Scotland told me that she had suffered from long COVID following a COVID-19 infection six months ago. When she mentioned "long COVID", I asked her whether she meant "already long COVID" or "still long COVID", or in other words whether she wanted to say that she had already been suffering from COVID-19 for a long time or that she was still suffering from COVID-19. I was in favour of us agreeing to call it "already long COVID". We might also call it "post-COVID syndrome", or in other words a "syndrome **following** COVID". She agreed with that.

She told me that she had been on sick leave for six months, with the exception of a brief period four months ago when she had unsuccessfully attempted to return to work. She suffered from chronic fatigue. Normally she was an active person who had plenty of energy all day long. She was an optimist with a positive attitude to life, who liked her job and was eager to take on new challenges. Previously she had been able to get by on seven hours of sleep. Now she needed 12 or 14 hours in order to function at all. Even after sleeping for all that time, she could only manage around two hours of activity. Then she'd need to rest for half an hour, and if she was lucky she might manage another two hours of activity.

I told her to ask the person who was so immensely tired to step out of her. She made the person sit on the sofa opposite, and described to me how she sagged down like a sack of potatoes. The woman herself involuntarily sat a little more upright, and seemed more alert. But she also looked extremely sad. I asked, "It seems to me that there's some sadness there. Would it be OK with you if the sad one inside you were to go and stand over there, next to the sofa?" The woman nodded and started to cry. "I don't know what's wrong with me. I never normally cry, and certainly not in front of other people. I'm a very strong person – and that's not just what I think, that's what all my friends and family say about me. Now you've made me cry!" "Let's imagine that there's several sad ones inside you. If you had to decide spontaneously, by picking a number out of thin air, how many might it be?" "Five or six." "Take a good look at them! How old are they? Do you have any idea of the kind of things that are making them so sad?" She told me that they included herself as a child, teenager, and adult. She had always been very independent. Her parents were affectionate and she got on well with them. But they had both always been very busy with work. The woman told me that she was always there for others but hardly ever asked for help in return, that no task was too much or too difficult when she was at work and that she took everything upon herself, but that her employer was also very demanding. Before she was signed off it had probably all been getting a bit much for her, but she was now better at setting boundaries.

While she was telling me about the life stories and attitudes of the sad ones who had been taken out of her, her movements and voice became more and more animated. Towards the end of the session, she told me that she felt more alert and healthier than she had at the start. During the following session, she reported that she could now manage three or four hours of activity after nine hours of sleep, and tackle more during this time than she had been able to before – not a breakthrough, but certainly an improvement.

8.5.2 Invisible friends

The following interventions combine the subtraction procedure and the addition procedure (as well as incorporating age regression and age progression). The persons are first dissociated from the client in each case, since they are associated with the problem, but then re-related to her as helper figures, since they may at the same time represent special resources for her. One example of this can be found under the heading, "The good mother in you – out of you – for you".[37] Other creative possibilities are set out below by way of illustration.

Two friends

I say something along the lines of the following to highly gifted children: "I have the impression that part of you is still playing in the sandpit and another part of you is holding debates with the philosophy dons at the university. There's not really much in common between you and others who are the same age as you. Might that be true?" I might continue as follows: "Situations like that aren't always much fun, but they're not really anything out of the ordinary for highly gifted children. At some point it all evens out. Imagine that the person who is playful like a small child were to step out of you and stand to the left of you, over there. Let's take a look at her: how is she standing? How does she look? Now imagine that the person who is already an adult, who likes thinking big thoughts about life and philosophising, were to step out of you and stand to the right of you. How does she look? These people are to the right and left of you, and you're in the middle. What feels different in you now?"

A 16-year-old told me that for the past few weeks she'd been panicking every time her parents left the house. She found it particularly difficult to be apart from her mother. It had started when her mother had gone back to work and the girl herself had picked up some after-school shifts in a supermarket. Her parents had never had much time for her because they were so busy with their jobs. She'd often been left alone with her sister, from as young an age as eight. I explained that maybe she needed to catch up on a bit of her childhood before she became fully grown, and to stock up on care and attention from her parents. She could tell her mother that there was no need to worry, but that the mother should make sure there was plenty of parental care on offer over the next few months while she was topping up her stocks. She could imagine the person who was already an adult stepping out of her and standing on her right, and the person who was still a child following and standing to her left. The teenager reported that the person on the right didn't need any more help from her, but the one on the left needed her protection. I invited her to show particular care to the latter, and asked whether the one on the right could also care for her. The teenager responded that the adult was more than able to take on that role, and that she could see the two of them having a great time with each other.

A 49-year-old woman explained that she could not stop dwelling on concerns about her changing hormone levels and doubts about whether she was still attractive and feminine, and that she had not yet found the right way of dealing with these worries. I suggested to her, "Imagine placing to the right of you the 'lovely old lady', the kind grandma who you will become, and look at her. Now imagine placing to the left of you the person who wants to continue to be pretty and desirable, and is indeed both of those things, someone who would catch any man's eye, and saying to her, 'You can stay with me for a while longer!' Look at them! You're standing in the middle between them. They're your friends. You don't need to decide between them. You can keep both of them with you. How do you feel about that?" The client beamed and said that she felt great about it.

8.5.3 Subtraction, addition, and transformation of real and potential persons

In keeping with the rule of "separate problems, link solutions", therapeutic modelling involves dissociating out of the client her internal image of the people she associates with the problem, and placing them in the room (subtraction). People who are associated with resources can be brought into the room and placed by her side (addition). The client can be invited to stand in their place and to experience how they (presumably) feel. A greeting can be used to ask her internal self to take anything that is helpful in terms of resources from here back to her starting place and to transport it over into her future life, or alternatively to the spaces occupied by other people "from her head" who need this resource (transformation).

The client (or an imagined clone of the client whom the client sends around the room) can carry the following types of information back and forth between the invisible persons and herself.

• Helpful information: the sceptic she was carrying around inside herself just now can be told how well the client is doing without her objections.

- State of mind: the lonely young girl she used to be (or the patient of today suffering burnout, or her strict father) can be filled up with the client's good experience towards the end of the session.

Only (strengthening) experiences that are associated with solutions are transferred.

(Weakening) experiences that are associated with problems are left in their respective places. Once the client has returned to her starting place, she can be told that the individual people who have been taken out of her will also change if they experience how she and the other people have filled themselves up with resources. The therapist can enquire about this positive change, thereby strengthening it in turn in the various dissociated persons and the client who is physically present.

There are a huge number of different ways in which internal images of real or possible persons can be dissociated from the client's ego experience, associated with this experience, dissociated within themselves, dissociated from each other, associated with each other, or transformed into other images. The following example demonstrates a number of possibilities.

The child on the windowsill

A 39-year-old women named Kerstin (not her real name) told me about her unfulfilled desire for children, about her failed attempts to get pregnant using assisted conception, and about how she felt torn between feelings of hope and giving up, sadness, paralysis, and a great many of other states of mind that seemed to contradict each other, and in some cases to lead to a total blockage of emotions. Her husband had a very optimistic temperament by nature and could handle the situation well, unlike her. Her objective for our work together was to "lighten up".

I invited her to take out of herself all of the Kerstins that we could distinguish, and to describe to me in more detail some of the more distinctive protagonists.

Then I asked her to place her husband next to her in her thoughts, and to place in the room as well the child who might perhaps come along one day or might perhaps not. She explained that the child was sitting on the windowsill and looking at her.

In view of the fact that a feeling of "lightening up" might be found in her husband, I asked her to go over to where her husband was standing in order to experience how he was feeling. She did so and burst out in violent sobs. She explained that she had had no idea how brave her husband was, and how much he had had to endure.

Once she had returned to her starting place, she told me that this had been a very valuable experience for her, since it had helped her to appreciate her husband's love and support even more.

Once again I asked her to describe the child on the windowsill to me; I asked her to send a greeting to her brain and to ask it to regulate all emotions and other bodily reactions in such a way as to benefit her, and invited her to sit in the same place as the child that had come from the future, from heaven or from a place where everything is possible.

She sat on the windowsill and swung her legs back and forth. When I asked what she (as the child of Kerstin) wanted to say to her parents, the child said that everything was absolutely fine, that they didn't need to worry so much and that everything would turn out OK.

I asked Kerstin to take with her everything that was worth taking from the child's experience and to return to her starting place. She sat there and swung her legs back and forth. When I asked what was different now, she described a remarkably effortless and carefree attitude to life.

How might her husband's demeanour change when he noticed this change in her? "He will also look relieved, free, and full of energy," she responded.

I asked her to go back again to where he was standing and to experience this.

She described the state to me from an internal perspective. I asked her to describe to me his external and internal attitude to his wife and to the child on the windowsill.

I wanted to know how the child would react after seeing that both parents were now so much happier. As I expected, the child felt even better. And what was it like for her, if she took her husband's place, to see the child even happier? Also even better ...

I asked her to take with her everything that she regarded as being worth taking, to return to her starting place and to tell me what else was now different. It was evident that she felt good. I wanted to know whether she realised that this feeling had come to stay. She said that she thought it would indeed stay. She asked whether there was anything I could do about the fact that she still felt "under pressure" somehow. We spoke about venting the heating system,[38] and she responded with satisfaction by saying that she now felt good. This marked the end of our work.[39]

8.5.4 Outside sofa and inside sofa

This is an intervention I use on a regular basis in couples therapy. A couple told me that they were dealing with a situation in which one partner was "responsible" for the activities that were more fun, that were perhaps also more respected by society and that typically took place "outside" the home, whereas the other carried out the inside tasks that were less fun and that were maybe less valued by society. In this situation, it is often the man who performs the "outside" tasks and the woman who performs the "inside" tasks; in rare cases, the roles are reversed. This is also a common area of conflict in gay and lesbian couples.[40]

1. In addition to the seats where the couple are currently sitting, the therapist also places two pairs of chairs opposite each other and refers to them as the "outside sofa" and the "inside sofa".
2. The therapist tells the man to take up a space on the "outside sofa", and tells the woman to sit diagonally opposite him on the "inside sofa". He asks both of them to describe their physical and mental experiences where they are sitting.
3. The therapist asks both partners to swap over and sit down in the space that is exactly opposite where they are now, or in other words for the woman to sit on

the "outside sofa" next to the space where her partner was previously sitting, and for the man to sit on the "inside sofa" next to the space where his wife was previously sitting. He asks both of them to provide feedback on what they notice in terms of emotions and physical well-being.

4. For a more in-depth approach, the therapist might ask the partners to sit down in the space where their partner was just sitting, so that they can experience in terms of bodily sensations how the partner might plausibly have felt while sitting there.

5. The therapist asks both of the partners to sit down together on the "outside sofa" and to talk about what they experience there. What are the advantages? Are there any disadvantages as well?

6. The therapist then asks both of the partners to sit down together on the "inside sofa" and to talk about what they experience there. What are the advantages? Are there any disadvantages as well?

7. If it appears helpful based on Steps 5 and 6, the therapist can ask both partners to go and sit on the "outside sofa" together again, to fill themselves up with what is good here, and then to stand up at the same time, walk over to the "inside sofa" and fill it up with what they have brought.

8. If the couple are happy to do so, he can also ask both of them to fill themselves up with the advantages of the "inside sofa" and to take this to the "outside sofa".

9. The therapist asks where the couple would like to sit while the exercise is being brought to a close. If finding an answer to this question is not a straightforward process, he should ask both of them to take with them everything helpful, to return to the sofa where they started and to look back on the process from there.

8.6 Therapeutic greetings

Therapeutic greetings[41] – a form of alert ultra-short hypnosis based on Ericksonian hypnotherapy – are another type of intervention. A distinction is made between dissociative, associative, transformative, and mixed greetings.

We'll start our exploration of this topic with an example. The aim being pursued is the stabilisation of therapeutic outcomes against sceptical authorities, or in other words potential objections by internal voices or external persons whose words might be assigned more weight by the client than those of the therapist.

The earth rotates forwards

"If I'm not mistaken, things are going much better for you now than before! Am I right? If so, give the following greeting to your brain: *this is here to stay!*

If there might in some sense be a person inside you who could have the slightest doubt that this is true, give him the following greeting: *what's new replaces what was there before.*

When you install a new operating system on your computer, you don't say, 'The computer might have been running the new operating system today, but that doesn't mean a thing – I'm sure that when it boots up tomorrow it'll be running Windows 97 again!'

When you install an app on your mobile phone, you don't say, 'That won't be there for long'. Instead, you quite rightly expect that it will stay there unless you get bored of it and uninstall it.

When you buy a car, you won't suddenly wake up to an empty garage tomorrow because the garage was empty for so long beforehand that the car has vanished into thin air. If a house is being built on the field next door, it doesn't suddenly start being deconstructed, brick by brick – it stays there, and new floors are added. When your neighbour tells you that his dog has died, you don't say to him, 'Well he's never been dead before, so I'm sure he'll be back again tomorrow!' The same would apply, of course, if the dog had puppies: they would still be there the day after tomorrow, and if the neighbour sold them, they'd be in the households that had bought them. They wouldn't disappear just because they hadn't been there before. Why should that be any different for you, if your internal self has found a new way of living that is better for it than how you have been living your life up until now?

Give the following greeting to your internal self: the earth always rotates forwards. *What you have discovered will stay with you.*[42]

It may however be the case – and tell your internal self this in the form of another greeting – *that it continues to develop*, in the same way that a bud develops into a blossom and the blossom turns into a fruit, which grows and grows and ripens and ripens."

The greeting, *"This is here to stay!"* is **associative** in nature, and links a resource experience with the ego and current experiences and with the experience of duration.[43]

The greeting is later strengthened as follows: *"What you have discovered will stay with you"*.

This greeting lends a synoptic meaning to the series of illustrative stories, and guides the client's attention back to the start.

The greeting, *"What's new replaces what was there before"* is **dissociative** in nature; it separates the helpful current experience from the unhelpful (symptomatic) previous experience, and thus the expectation (the "future") from the memory (the "past"). This means that the old cycle of memory, expectation, and experience is interrupted, and a new cycle is initiated in which expectation is based not on memories that were experienced intensively (trauma) or for a long time (chronic stress) or often (recurrent stress), but instead on what is currently being experienced (therapeutic effect). The implication that what exists now is identical to what is coming (expectation, future) is incorporated as an aspect of an associative greeting.

The choice of these interventions at this point adheres to the following rule: "The fewer the client's objections to the therapy at the end of the session, the more stable the outcome."[44] The additional examples serve to establish plausibility through vividness (perceptibility). Switching between different examples helps to forestall from the outset any debates concerning the transferability of these examples. The wide range of examples also creates the impression that this is a universal law that is all the less likely to be potentially called into question.

The greeting, *"that it continues to develop"* is of a **transformative** nature. The client is presented with images illustrating the concept that what has already been achieved will develop further in a valuable and at the same time unavoidable fashion. It is implied that the good will remain and expand all on its own.

8.6.1 Dissociative greetings

I often use dissociative greetings in trauma therapy, but also with individuals suffering from allergies who have come to therapy. In this case it is useful for people to be able to recollect earlier times in their life when they reacted allergically, without at the same time exhibiting the start of an allergic reaction which might – akin to a panic spiral – involuntarily turn into a full-scale allergic reaction.

Decoupling physical memory and film memory

I use the following greeting when people start to talk about potentially traumatic experiences during a therapy session, or if I suspect that the course of the conversation might lead there.

"You can view images of how it was previously, but without experiencing the previous bodily reactions and emotions. In order to allow this to happen, your internal self detaches the film memory from the physical memory, so that you can have one without the other. Tell your body that it should make sure that this happens, both during our work and beyond that!"

8.6.2 Associative greetings

The following greeting creates an associative connection in the brain that was not there beforehand. I use it during therapy sessions with individuals suffering from sleep apnoea.

At the first indications (preconscious anchors)

"Give a greeting to your body, and tell it that at the *first indication* of a hesitation in your breathing during the night it should take a particularly deep breath, so that you can continue sleeping and your sleep will be all the more pleasant."[45]

A similar procedure can be used with clients who have trouble remaining asleep all night, for example due to depression or grief. The therapist tells his client to send a message to his body saying that from now on, at the first indications of any such waking, it should go into a deeper and ever deeper sleep, instead of waking up like before.[46]

8.6.3 Transformative greetings

Below is an example of a transformative greeting, or in other words a short intervention aimed at transforming, in gradual transitions, a stressful experience or an experience that generates complications into a less symptomatic experience or an experience associated with solutions.

This frequently takes place using the visual imagination, or in other words with internal films. A transformation from acoustic (verbal language or sound) or physical and emotional experiences is, however, also possible, in which case physical symptoms are transformed into emotions. The procedure has proven successful for a very large number of symptoms, including various skin disorders.[47]

Transforming symptoms into emotions I

During the two days after being vaccinated against COVID-19 for the first time, I felt dizzy, nauseous, and fatigued, and I also suffered from headaches and a brief but extremely violent bout of chills. When I was vaccinated for the second time, two doctors told me that I should expect a severe reaction. I would probably have flu-like symptoms for two or three days. In my head, I said to my body, "Please transform any symptom of which there is even the slightest trace into an emotion." Sometimes I felt a slight sweat breaking out, a small amount of fatigue or the very first signs of a headache or dizziness, as well as a barely perceptible burning sensation at the vaccination site. If I hadn't been paying attention, I probably wouldn't have noticed any of it at all. On several occasions I experienced waves of sadness, but these passed as quickly as they had come. I repeated the procedure when I was vaccinated for the third time. This time the sadness was even more pronounced and I noticed almost no physical symptoms at all – which was a reaction I was more than happy with. My sadness centred around illnesses I had experienced earlier that had led me to be categorised as clinically extremely vulnerable during the COVID-19 pandemic.[48]

I'd suggest the following to anyone else getting vaccinated: "Give your internal self a greeting and tell it that it should transform every symptom that might arise as a vaccine reaction into an emotion, preconsciously and involuntarily! These emotions might be sadness or annoyance, melancholy or loneliness. If you like, you can monitor which emotions come along, and what they remind you of."

Erickson was also familiar with methods for converting symptoms into emotions using only a few words. Once a woman suffering from psoriasis came to see him. He looked at the affected area, and said, "You haven't got more than one-third of the psoriasis that you think you have … You've got a little psoriasis and a lot of emotions." The woman was angry with him for two weeks, until she noticed that the psoriasis had disappeared.[49]

8.6.4 Mixed greetings

Many greetings involve presenting a mixture of dissociative, associative, and transformative suggestions. Here are two examples of greetings for clients who start talking about experiences that appear to have had a traumatic effect on them.

Nothing gets the upper hand

"Can we reach an agreement with your mind that whatever paths we might follow, nothing – no emotion and no bodily reaction – will ever get the upper hand (**dissociative**), but that your mind will guide you back to well-being again and again (**associative**) and regulate everything just as it should be (**transformative**)?"

Thinking calmly about bad things

"Tell your brain that it should ensure that you can also think about things that up until now (**dissociative with reference to the past**) could have been extremely unpleasant (**dissociative with reference to reality**), and that you can do so with remarkable calm and serenity (**associative**)! Your brain can do that."[50]

8.7 Therapeutic rituals

In keeping with the principle that, "the more perceptible the therapy, the more effective it is",[51] objects and actions with a symbolic meaning can clarify what is to happen in therapy. The memory becomes more intense (and is therefore perceived to be more relevant) as a result of the increased clarity; this serves as a basis for new expectations, from which future experience is formed.

> Rituals are concentrated sequences that are repeated in the sense of a condensed, collective and symbolic action. As such, they form part of the traditions handed down by all cultures, and may in fact also represent the oldest form of psychotherapy ... In some respects, psychotherapy itself is also a type of ritual, which allows clients to achieve a change in status from problem state to non-problem state and provides a framework for this purpose ...[52]

8.7.1 Technical rituals

Technical metaphors can translate very effectively into representational symbols and action-focused rituals.

Defrosting the fridge

A woman came to see me and said she was seeking a sex therapist. In response to the question of why she wanted me to act as her therapist, she said, "You work in the tradition of Milton Erickson, don't you? He once had a woman come to him and tell him that she was frigid. He sent her home with the task of defrosting her fridge. It helped her. When I heard this story, I realised that I wanted a therapist like that as well."[53]

A reader asked whether this was a ritual. If it was intended to improve the technical operation and hygiene of the appliance, probably not. If it was intended as a medical prescription to be followed in order to promote healing, perhaps. I would interpret it as a threshold ritual that differentiates the old from the new, and marks the transition into a new state by means of a symbolic action. It is the context that makes the difference in this case.

Oiling the door handle

Metaphors that are enacted and can therefore be experienced physically (*enacted* or *living metaphors*)[54] can also be used *within* a therapy session. A doctor once told me the following story.

> I once treated a woman who suffered from arthritis in her thumbs. She had seen a lot of improvement in one thumb after taking some herbal medicine made from devil's claw, but it was still very difficult to move the other thumb, which hurt every time she tried. I gave her a homeopathic injection, and walked with her to the door so that we could say our goodbyes. The door handle creaked terribly. It had been like that for a long time, but this time it bothered me for some reason. I grabbed some WD40 for the hinge while we were still chatting. I sprayed it on and moved the door handle back and forth several times. While I was busy doing that, I noticed that the woman was also moving her thumb back and forth at the same time. This fascinated me. "Look, your thumb is just like the door handle," I said. Then I moved the door handle again, and said, "Now it's not creaking any more." "Yes, and now my thumb isn't hurting any more," replied the woman, moving her thumb back and forth.[55]

8.7.2 Care rituals

Care for pets, houseplants, or a piece of nature in the great outdoors can be an illustrative model of good self-care, of a home country, or of belonging, or in other words the ability to be connected to others in a reciprocal relationship of giving and taking, and the confidence to live in the expectation of a long life that is worth living.

Turning shit into roses

There are various different versions of this ritual. The first example relates to a woman who did more for others than for herself, and also held others in much higher regard than herself; the second relates to a 10-year-old boy who soiled himself (encopresis).

"I always put my needs last after those of everyone else, and I think that everything I do is shit, so when others treat me like shit, it seems to me like they're right to do so!" said a colleague.

"I think that you are indeed a rose. Although we might not agree on that point," I answered. "Do you know what skatole is?" "No." "It's an aromatic substance that is used in the perfume industry. Skatole is what makes roses smell like roses. But it's also precisely what makes shit smell like shit.[56] It depends on the concentration. In the USA they talk about, 'turning shit into roses.'[57] Do you have a garden?" "Yes. And there's even a large rose bush in it!" "I have a task for you. Buy a sack of manure, guano, or something else that contains shit. Fertilise your roses with it and see what happens then!"

Two years later the colleague referred back to the conversation in an email, and said that it had benefited her, "to be able to fertilise my rose bush, and to be able to receive its gratitude in the form of beautiful bright white flowers".

The mother who drew a map of the guano islands together with her son[58] told me some time later that the soiling problem had got much better, but had not yet gone away entirely. I asked her to take the boy to the garden centre and to buy a sack of guano fertiliser and two houseplants. They should fertilise one of the plants with guano, and leave the other one alone. Both should be placed on the windowsill in the boy's room, and they should water them regularly together. A little while later the mother reported that she and her son had bought three plants that looked roughly the same. One was given only water, the second a brew of dandelions and red currants which the boy wanted to try, and the third guano. A few weeks later the first plant had died, the second had survived and the third had blossomed. During this period the young boy stopped soiling himself.

8.7.3 Rituals of farewell and new beginnings

Rituals of farewell and new beginnings can help clients to find their role and identity in a new stage of life, to disentangle mixtures of sadness and beauty, to set boundaries around themselves and to experience belonging across space, time, and even the threshold of death.

Cutting the umbilical cord

I've used this ritual several times with women who told me that they had "not yet cut the umbilical cord", or in other words when talk turned to the topic of detaching from their mother. Here is one example.

"My mother's 82, but she's in great shape for her age. The problem is that she moans a lot, and I always end up giving in and doing whatever she wants me to do. I feel like there's no point though, because afterwards she moans just as much. I'm annoyed with myself for being so dependent on her. Somehow I haven't quite managed to cut the umbilical cord yet."

"Wait one second," I answered, left the room and returned a few minutes later with a number of utensils – or, to be more precise, with a pair of scissors, a piece of cord, and two clothes pegs. I clipped the clothes pegs to the cord, which I laid over my knees. "Who should cut the umbilical cord – would you like to do it, or shall I? Or shall I do it acting as your mother?" I put the scissors to the cord, waited a moment and then cut it. The client took a few deep breaths, as though something pivotal had happened. She was visibly moved, and her voice sounded emotional when she told me that the ritual had "shifted something around inside her", and that she felt different.

During the next session she said that this ritual had changed her internal attitude towards her mother, and that she felt freer.

I have carried out a similar ritual twice more in similar situations with other clients: once in a face-to-face session, and once during a video call. Each time the effect was remarkable.

Swapping the native soil

I use rituals described below in courses of therapy where migration or grief (or sometimes a combination of both) play a central role.

I suggested the following to an immigrant suffering from home sickness: "The next time you visit your relatives in Russia, remove a handful of soil from your garden here and take it to a garden there that you love. Talk to the soil and give it your blessing, so that it helps the plants and animals living on it to thrive. Then remove a handful of soil from there and bring it to Germany, and place it either in your garden or a flowerpot in your kitchen. Give this soil a blessing as well, so that it helps things to thrive. If you like, you can plant something in it, water it, and watch how it grows."

In another situation I asked a woman to bring a flower from home and to place it on the grave of a person she had loved who was buried a long way away. Conversely, she could bring home with her a stone, a small amount of soil, or a plant from their grave, and set up a small shrine in her home with it.

Re-consecration

I have initiated rituals similar to the one described below if a client is torn between longing for an ex-partner and anger at him, and – despite this conflicted emotional state – continues to live in a house where everything reminds her of her ex.

"Every picture, every wall, every piece of furniture in the house reminds me of my ex-husband. I'd like to forget him and move on with my life, but everything reminds me of him, and there are practical and financial reasons why I can't move house."

"I have one request for you: buy a spray bottle, one of the ones with an atomiser. Fill it up with water. Ask the people you love and who are important to you to come over for the afternoon or evening, and give them a small piece of absorbent paper. Ask them to write a blessing or some kind words for you on the paper, and to give it back to you again. You'll also need to buy some essential oil with a smell that you love. Put a few drops of this oil on each piece of paper. Then place the pieces of paper in the spray bottle and give it a good shake. Now walk together through the house and re-consecrate it. Perhaps one of your friends can play a musical instrument or sing at the same time. Or you can hand out saucepan lids so that people can bang and crash and make such a loud noise together that you drive out the spirits of the past. Take the bottle and spray the whole house with it, every single room."

8.7.4 Healing rituals

Healing rituals can help to make perceptible the body's capacities for regulating and regenerating itself, and sometimes reduce or heal symptoms and diseases rapidly and permanently in the process.

Pulling symptoms out of the body

"May I try pulling that out of you?" I sometimes say to people with neck or back pain or who are suffering from tension or discomfort, including in the neck or back area, while I reach out my arm in their direction as though I wanted to grab onto something. I wait – with an amicable mixture of seriousness and humour – until I receive a nod of the head or a "yes" from them. Then I make a performance of pulling something out of their back, as though I were pulling a fishing net out of the sea. Gradually the movements become less and less exaggerated, until the very last bit of whatever it is has been removed from their back with a small jerk. Sometimes I heighten the effect with panting noises and a look of anguished exertion. Other times I wrap whatever has come out of their back around my arm, around an imaginary cable winch, or on a cable drum, and often I throw it directly onto the floor in front of the client. I generally ask them to describe what is lying there in terms of its material, structure, and colour. Then I ask how their back is feeling. "Much better! But I can still just feel a little twinge ..." is the most common answer. And so I repeat the procedure another three, four, five, or six times. The colour and often also the material and structure of whatever has been removed vary, and detailed enquiries reveal that the residual symptoms that remain in each case are also not exactly the same as they were before. They have become weaker, feel different, have shifted from the centre of the region that was previously symptomatic to its edges, etc.

On several occasions I have pulled tinnitus sounds "out of clients' ears" as beams or threads. We had previously discussed what the sounds might look like if they were visible. I have carried out many such interventions during video calls. I suggested to clients that, "if you don't mind, I'll just reach over through the screen and pull it out", which interestingly enough was accepted without discussion.

In the case of clients who find physical closeness and unconventional forms of treatment unproblematic, I sometimes ask for permission to "pull out of them" a headache or heaviness behind the eyes. I place a hand on the affected part of the body and pull, as though I wanted to pull plasticine or a slimy substance out of their head. Sometimes I ask them to help by sending the pain into my hand. Afterwards I shake my hand vigorously with an expression of horror and aversion. Then I ask how they are now feeling, and repeat different versions of the procedure if necessary. Based on the feedback I have received, the symptom-reducing effect of the procedure is perceptible to a significant degree.

What I stroke

This ritual, which has been handed down as folk medicine, is used for warts, different skin conditions, and internal diseases, among other things.

The experiments I have conducted lead me to believe that it generally works.

I assume that there are no scientific studies into its effectiveness.

Individuals with warts can be asked to perform an ancient ritual. It stems from the repertoire of the "*Braucher*", or in other words women (or in rare instances men) who are learned in the magical and religious customs of the folk medicine that can be traced back to shamanic traditions in the Central European region. I learned it from an old healer who said that she herself had learned it in her youth from an old woman in Bavaria, where it has been practised by some families for generations, and is also used for internal complaints.

The person with the wart is supposed to lick their index finger, stroke it over the wart in a circular fashion and say out loud, "What I stroke, take away!" They should carry out the procedure again with the middle finger and ring finger, and repeat the whole thing three times daily until the wart has disappeared. Another form of the saying is as follows: "What I behold, may it vanish, and what I stroke, may it melt."[59] Yet another regional form of the ritual takes the following form: when the moon is waxing, the individual wanting to get rid of a wart should look at the night sky on a daily (or nightly) basis, stroke the wart and say, "What I behold, may it increase. What I stroke, may it decrease."[60]

The interesting thing about this last version of the ritual is that it picks up on the ambivalence of symptoms; if they were not beneficial in some way or if they did not at least have a good intention, they would not come into being or persist. Yet if they were wanted, there would be no need to get rid of them.[61] This ambivalence or double bind is dissociated in a therapeutic counter double bind: the desire to increase and to remain is coupled with the moon and thereby decoupled vividly and plausibly from the wart, and the desire to reduce is linked to the wart.[62]

I initially tried out the method myself several times to treat warts and lipomas,[63] and then recommended it to others. It took between three days and two weeks of treatment until the problem had completely vanished, or three weeks in the case of a plantar wart on the sole of the foot. In one case we translated the rhyme into French, but once again the outcome was entirely satisfactory.

Warts are also "talked over"[64] in hypnotherapy, with the difference that "suggestion" is the underlying healing principle rather than a spiritual world.

Laying on of hands

In a secularised society, rituals such as the laying on of hands, faith healing, and blessings are not necessarily an easy sell. They do not match up with what people generally expect of a psychotherapist, doctor, or coach. This says nothing about the potential effectiveness of rituals of this kind, but a lot about expectations of roles, or in other words the possibility of achieving successful therapeutic outcomes through good pacing. Such rituals can, however, be appropriate for preschool children or individuals with Christian beliefs. It's also possible to render these rituals newly plausible and therefore beneficial for the modern era …

The therapist can say to the client,

"A trauma or a conflict is often particularly stressful if there is no one there to support us during this period. At some point you decide to ignore the problem and try and forget about it. But sometimes it then tries to find a place for itself in your body, for example somewhere that has always been a weak spot for you or somewhere with symbolic meaning. I'm not sure whether you'd call it a home or a prison. It settles down there and produces symptoms, sometimes for years or decades, until someone shows some care and attention to the problem and its needs. Trauma is a combination of powerlessness and loneliness, and conflicts involve not being able to get vital needs met because getting other needs met runs counter to this goal.

"If it's OK with you, I'd like to try something unusual. May I lay my hand over the part of your body that has not wanted to heal up until now? Imagine that this hand is a heat lamp emitting welcome and acceptance, love and respect, what you were missing during the time when the symptom first emerged, or even beforehand, perhaps as a small child, perhaps even what your parents and ancestors were missing, who knows. If I may, let's summon this warmth, this welcome and this respect for your dignity like a blessing from the world of love, so that it can find a home in your body, where it is needed: from the invisible world where love resides, we summon this flow of warmth to this point in your body where something has established itself, something like suppressed anger or grief or loneliness or fear … more and more … more and more … more and more … What has changed now?"

The therapist generates plausibility for the procedure's effectiveness by referring to the principle that was described as No. 6 of the "factors affecting therapy".[65] The intuitively perceived plausibility connected with this ancient ritual undoubtedly also has an impact. Mechanisms of action that would require spiritual rather than psychobiological words to describe them should be neither disputed nor speculatively asserted at this point.

During video calls, the therapist can say, "If it's OK with you, I'll lay my hand on this part of your body," and perform the gesture in the form of a mime. "In your mind, sense how my hand is resting there. Can you feel that?"

Another example of the laying on of hands in therapeutic work is described above under the heading "Pulling symptoms out of the body".

Transforming symptoms into emotions II

A participant in a video seminar told me that she had caught COVID-19. She already felt a lot better, but was still suffering from headaches, a sore throat, a hoarse voice, and a feeling of permanent exhaustion. She was also sweating excessively, and sometimes had a temperature.

I asked her to imagine transforming the headaches into an emotion and feeling this emotion. What had happened to her pain now? It had lessened greatly, and there was only a certain amount of pressure left. I asked her to transform this pressure into an emotion as well, and to feel it. Then I asked her to transform the exhaustion into an emotion or something similar, and to tell me what she felt. After that I asked her to transform the sore throat and hoarse voice into emotions, and to feel what they were like. Finally, I asked her to transform the sweating and raised body temperature into emotions and to feel these.

From time to time, I would intersperse questions about the issues, individuals, and events from the past few weeks or months with which she associated the emotional reactions, and discussions ensued about the stressful situations that had bothered her recently.

I asked the participant what symptoms she still had.

"None," she answered, with an incredulous and astonished expression. When I asked her again after half a day and once again after a whole day, she confirmed that the symptoms had stayed away.

The effectiveness of the procedure is based on Factor 6 mentioned in the second Chapter.[66]

Another participant in the same seminar had reacted badly after receiving a COVID-19 vaccine. The same procedure, with the addition of steps for removing the persons within her who experienced headaches, chills, arm pain etc. (or in other words the subtraction procedure from therapeutic modelling), meant that she too was free of symptoms within a short space of time, and this continued to be the case when the seminar ended two days later.

It is possible that the huge variations in the symptoms experienced by individuals infected with COVID-19 and the varying severity of vaccine reactions can partially be explained by predispositions associated with biographical experiences.

Notes

1   Hammel 2019a, 124, Hammel 2014a, 68 et seqq.
2   A further order-related metaphor can be found in Chapter 3, Section "Role and identity"/"Perpetrators and victims" under the heading "strawberry mash and manure".
3   We also discussed the dilation of blood vessels and the body's ability to regulate blood pressure differently in the various parts of the body. This resulted in the problem being worked through to the woman's complete satisfaction.
4   It is similarly possible to talk about filters or valves with certain clients (cf. Hammel 2012c, 49), about pressure cookers or steam engines with others who suffer from high blood pressure and are clearly overworking themselves (see Hammel 2019a, 35 et seq.) or about process engineering system\s for separating emulsions with people who have suffered intra-family trauma (see Hammel 2016a, 53).
5   See the intervention "Oiling the door handle" in Chapter 8, Section "Therapeutic rituals"/"Technical rituals".
6   Hammel et al. 2018, 55.
7   The metaphor can also be used for allergies and other autoimmune diseases. The same narrative pattern can be found in the story "Civil war and civil peace" in Hammel 2012c, 49 et seq.
8   See Section "Therapeutic stories"/"Shared life experience" in this chapter.
9   See Hammel 2020, 81 et seq.
10   Hammel 2020, 53.
11   Some of the following passages are taken from Hammel et al. 2020, 124 et seqq.
12   Techniques for the spontaneous development of stories can be found in Hammel 2019a, 209 et seqq., passim.
13   For structures that can be used to build stories of this kind, see ibid. 300 et seqq.
14   See Chapter 2, Section "Therapeutic maps and landscapes"/"Idiomatic landscapes".
15   See the story "Barbarossa" under the heading "Shared life experience" further down in this chapter and section. Another example of a more metaphorical negative learning model is "The tribe of the clueless" in Hammel 2011, 125. Confrontational illustrative stories that are not always suitable in therapy include: "Tomorrow" (Hammel 2012c, 51) and "What God has joined together". See ibid., 63 et seq.
16   For further details of changes in punctuation, see Watzlawick et al. 2011, 18, 141.
17   Based on Hammel 2019a, 63 et seq.
18   Hammel 2011, 118 et seq.
19   See Chapter 6, Section on hypnotherapy, ""Factors affecting therapy", Factor 6.
20   See Section "Therapeutic rituals"/"Healing rituals" in this chapter.
21   Based on Hammel 2019a, 176, with original quotes from my Year 1 and Year 2 reports.
22   Hammel et al. 2018, 91 et seq. The following have a similar structure: "Gregor the dragon" in Hammel 2019a, 172 et seq.; "Of the extinction of the dragon killers" in Hammel et al. 2021, 102 et seq.; "The dance of the unicorns" in Hammel 2016b, 45 et seqq.
23   I.e., using "The Island of Love" map or self-produced island maps.
24   Another therapy session in which the "guano islands" were used as an intervention with a child suffering from encopresis can be found in Hammel 2014a, 166 et seqq.
25   For a discussion of the initial situation and the therapeutic procedure, see Hammel 2019a, 131 et seq.

26 Rules-based logic and exception-based logic can also be amalgamated in the form of "documentary film logic". For further details of working with metaphors in accordance with a rules-based, exception-based or cartoon-based logic, see Hammel 2012c, 155 et seqq. and Hammel 2019a, 210 *et seqq.*

27 And vice versa; for Ina Hullmann, the "island of understanding", which represents a constricted perception of the problem experience, is surrounded by the "ocean of possibilities", representing an expanded perception with humorous and compassionate levity. See Hullmann 2020, 5 et seq.

28 The intervention "Mountain village" is a more detailed variant of this method. Another example for the method of altering imagined landscapes using the documentary film technique, is found in Hammel 2012c, 73.

29 For further details of the methodology for transforming imagined landscapes that depict the described life situation using the cartoon technique or the superimposition technique, see Hammel 2012c, 57, 128 et seq.; Hammel 2019a, 214. Ortwin Meiss has developed a similar procedure in his work with hypnosystemic therapy, see Meiss 2016, 206.

30 See Chapter 2, section on hypnotherapy, "Factors affecting therapy", Factor 1.

31 Timeline work can probably be attributed to Tad James or Richard Bandler, or possibly to a counselling technique that existed beforehand, see www.nlpportal.org/nlpedia/wiki/Time_Line.

32 The method is outlined here through the lens of my experience and interpretation, merely as a prompt for further ideas, and should not be interpreted as an attempt to reproduce Nemetschek's model on a one-to-one basis. It follows that certain elements have been abbreviated, whereas others have been altered and developed further to reflect my practice. Nemetschek presents his model in Holtz et al. 2000, 114 et seqq. as well as in Nemetschek 2006, 96 et seqq. A wide range of variants for individual and team coaching sessions can be found in Theureutzbacher & Nemetschek 2009. The diagram "Standard 'river of life'" work at the end of this section is taken from Nemetschek 2006, 104.

33 I learned this procedure from Birgit Steiner-Backhausen. It is probably based on one of the NLP formats using floor anchors ("collapsing anchors" or "change history"), see www.nlpportal.org/nlpedia/wiki/Collapsing_Anchors and www.nlpportal.org/nlpedia/wiki/Change_History.

34 Once again, the following applies: the model is reproduced through the filter of my experience and interpretation. As a result, certain elements are represented in abbreviated form, whereas others have developed further in my practice. A detailed account of the model and its potential applications can be found in Varga von Kibéd & Sparrer 2000, 75 et seqq.

35 The phenomenon can be viewed in various places, e.g. at www.entdeckerlab.de/blog/zuendholz-gleichgewicht-experiment.

36 Many different examples of working with the therapeutic modelling method can be found in Chapter 2, Section "Assumptions and attitudes from psychodrama, constellation work and parts work" as well as in Chapter 7, Section "History-taking using life opportunities". Detailed descriptions of this approach can be found in Hammel 2019b and Hammel et al. 2020, 74. For further details of couples therapy using therapeutic modelling, see Kolodej 2016, 175 et seqq.; Hammel 2014b and Hammel 2019b, 105 et seqq., 205 et seqq. and 260 et seqq.

37 See Chapter 3, Section "Role and identity"/"New allegiances".

38 See "Bleeding the radiators" in Chapter 9, "Conclusion and following session"/"Dispelling doubts and building optimism".

39 The procedure of switching between various real or imagined (possible) persons, allowing the advantages of each position to benefit the other persons and increasing this well-being in a circular fashion, is used in connection with exam nerves in Hammel

et al. 2020, 78 et seqq. Two years after the session the woman gave birth to a child conceived naturally and claimed that it was "the one who sat on the windowsill".

40 The hints and tips provided in the introduction to Section "Therapeutic modelling" in this chapter should be observed if the work is being carried out during a video call.

41 A detailed description of the way in which therapeutic greetings work together with many examples of the methodology can be found in Hammel 2020.

42 "The balance wheel" in Hammel et al. 2015, 77 et seq. is a similarly structured intervention.

43 See Figure 2.3 "Separate problems, link solutions" in Chapter 2, section on hypnotherapy ("Separating, linking, and transforming").

44 See Chapter 2, section on hypnotherapy, "Factors affecting therapy", Factor 3. Interruptions to the cycle of memory, expectation, and experience are discussed in the same chapter and section under the heading "The cycle of memory and expectation" as well as in Chapter 9.

45 See Hammel 2020, 63.

46 Ibid., 62.

47 Case studies relating to the transformation of symptoms into emotions using other therapeutic techniques can be found at the end of this chapter ("Healing rituals"). Additional transformative greetings can be found at the end of the story "Storm at sea and the polar ocean" in Chapter 3 ("The ambivalence of pain and numbness"), in the case study "The child on the windowsill" in this chapter ("Therapeutic modelling"/"Subtraction, addition, and transformation...") and in the intervention "Announcing the unconscious effects of practice" in Chapter 9, ("Feedback on developments...").

48 I first received the Astra Zeneca vaccine; three months later I received the Biontech/Pfizer vaccine, and six months after that the Biontech/Pfizer vaccine again.

49 Rosen 1982, 154 et seq. The procedure followed in the aforesaid cases is based on applying the principle underlying Factor 6 in Chapter 2, section on hypnotherapy, "Factors affecting therapy".

50 See Hammel 2020, 36 et seq. (emphases in brackets added secondarily).

51 Factor 1 in Chapter 2, section on hypnotherapy, "Factors affecting therapy".

52 Schlippe & Schweitzer 1996, 190.

53 I can certainly believe that this is something that Erickson would have said, but I have been unable to find a source for it despite exhaustive investigations.

54 Hammel 2012c, 154 et seq.; Hammel 2019a, 287 et seq.

55 Hammel 2011, 60.

56 "Skatole is the primary contributor to faecal odour ... When highly diluted, skatole has a pure scent of roses that is low in secondary aromas, and is used in trace amounts in the perfumery industry", https://de.wikipedia.org/wiki/Skatol.

57 The idiom was originally, "fall into shit and come up smelling like roses", but today it is mostly abbreviated to, "come up smelling like roses". Another version is, "turn shit into roses".

58 See Section "Therapeutic maps and landscapes"/"Self-produced island maps".

59 Herz 2010, 66. The latter also contains additional prayers and rituals for treating warts in keeping with this tradition. Within the German-speaking countries, remnants of this custom can still be found in the Alpine regions (among others).

60 This version is based on what I was told by another seminar participant whose (predominantly rural) family had passed down the ritual in this form over several generations.

61 See the discussion in Chapter 3, section "Ambivalence and conflict"/"Problems as ambivalences".

62 This fits in with Paul Watzlawick's view that opposites in systems balance each other out and stabilise each other (first-order system: human body with wart). It is possible to bring about the wholesale disintegration of stable states within a system of this kind if a

solution is found that is based not within the relevant system (body), but instead within a hierarchically superior system (second-order system: earth with moon as the surroundings of the human). Watzlawick et al. 2011, 75 *et seqq.*

63 See Hammel 2019a, 47 et seq.
64 Olness & Kohen 2011, 264 et seqq.; Hammond 1990, 223 et seqq.
65 See Chapter 2, section on hypnotherapy.
66 Section on hypnotherapy, "Factors affecting therapy".

Chapter 9

Conclusion and following session

When the session is drawing to a close, the therapist can guide the client's attention towards what has been achieved and what the next steps should be:

- What has been achieved in terms of the client's objectives for the session?
- What (if anything) still needs to be done?
- Which new objectives (if any) have been brought into focus?
- What are the client's questions or concerns (if any) about the outcome?
- Is there a need for something to protect what has been achieved against internal doubts and the scepticism of other influential people within the client's system?
- Are there any rituals, exercises, or tasks that the client can use to consolidate the outcome of the session?
- Does the client have any resolutions that she would like to act on by the next session, and should any firm commitments be undertaken in this respect?
- What kind of agreement should be reached with regard to any future therapy sessions?

9.1 Dispelling doubts and building optimism

Before a session ends, it is important to ensure that the client is contemplating the future with optimism and that any doubts about the effectiveness and long-lasting nature of the work are dispelled to the maximum extent possible. Concerns and objections function as counter-suggestions to the content of the therapeutic suggestion, since they generate an opposing expectation, and expectations tend to implement themselves as experiences (which become memories, which become expectations …).[1]

What can we do to confirm clients in their belief that the outcomes of therapy are long-lasting and that their problems will therefore be solved for good?

The "right now" box and the "always" box (the "would be" box and the "is" box)

I regularly encounter clients who say something along the lines of the following towards the end of a session: "Right now I feel great. But I don't know whether that feeling will last." Sometimes I give the following answer.

DOI: 10.4324/9781003425014-12

"There are two concepts of time. One says that the present is an infinitely brief point in time, sandwiched between the past and the future, and the other says that the present is eternal because it is always 'now', after all. Similarly, we have two words for the present. Sometimes we say 'right now' and sometimes we say 'always'. Strangely enough, people mostly say 'right now' for the good things in life, and 'always' for the bad things. When viewed from the perspective of suggestions and self-fulfilling prophecies, it's a much better idea to switch them around.

Imagine that you have two boxes in your mind: the 'right now' box and the 'always' box. Ask your mind to swap the content of these two boxes. Then we'd have to change what you just said to the following: 'I feel great, and I'll always feel great until the opposite is proven, if it ever is.' What do you think?"

If clients say, "It would be nice if it stayed like that," the intervention looks like this.

"There are two boxes in your mind. The 'would be' box and the 'is' box. What ends up in the 'would be' box and what ends up in the 'is' box typically has nothing to do with whether an event is likely or unlikely. Instead, people normally put the nice things in the 'would be' box so that they're not disappointed if they don't stick around, and the less nice things in the 'is' box so that they're not disappointed if they stay. But it's a much better idea to do it the other way around. Try telling your mind that it should swap the contents of the boxes. Then what you just said would sound like this: 'It's nice if it stays like that,' or perhaps even, 'It's nice like that'. Could we also put it like that?"

The journey to the "would be" planet

"The journey to the 'would be' planet" is similar to swapping the contents of the "would be" box and the "is" box in certain respects, but is also reminiscent of the miracle question. From a hypnotherapeutic perspective, it involves the induction of a trance through the generation of confusion (confusion induction). I sometimes use this intervention during the phase of clarifying objectives, if clients respond to the following question: "Supposing we achieve the best possible outcome today, what will have changed?" with the response, "It would be nice if I could … (XYZ)."

Imagine there are two planets: the "would be" planet and the "is" planet. You're currently living on the "is" planet. It's nicer on the "would be" planet, where things are as they would be if things were going well. Imagine that there's a shuttle service between the two planets. You can commute between them in a spaceship. Imagine travelling through space and landing on the "would be" planet. It has a pleasant climate and good living conditions. But the people who live on the "would be" planet don't see themselves as "would be" people in the slightest. They say, "things here are like they are here, and things on your planet would be like they would be with you." They call their planet the "is" planet and our planet, the planet you come from, the "would be" planet. And once you've lived on their planet for a while, you can understand what they mean, and you say, "Previously I thought it *would be* here. But it *is* here, and it would be where I previously was if I went there again ... Is that making sense to you?"

On the side turned towards me

I sometimes also tell the following story to clients that express ideas of this kind. "After a car trip through Lüneburg Heath, a physicist from Göttingen was asked by friends whether the sheep there had already been shorn. His answer was as follows: 'Not on the side turned towards me.'"[2]

This anecdote uses a therapeutic double bind. The sceptic's scientific accuracy is positively highlighted, and the irrelevance of his answer in terms of rural life is humorously turned into a joke. The narrative context implies that the client's scepticism likewise creates objections that are logically accurate but irrelevant in practice. The intervention produces an effect regardless of whether clients are aware of the story's intention.

Ministerial posts

Following a therapeutic modelling approach, we could take the person who has objections out of the client (**subtraction**), honour her good intentions and put them to better use elsewhere, for example by suggesting that she – who only wanted to protect the client against disappointment, but in the process insinuated a self-fulfilling prophecy – should take up a post as Minister for Confidence and Optimism in the client's life (**transformation**), ask her in a ceremonial manner, "Do you accept the post?", and ask the client what she answers.[3] If further objections emerge during the course of the conversation, we can also appoint these naysayers as dignitaries and offer them posts as secretaries of state within the Ministry of Confidence and Optimism. Positions, including head of department, advisor, clerk, trainee, and intern, can be assigned during further rounds of the procedure. Alternatively, the "person who likes to be in control" can be named the "Minister for Belonging, Home, and Herd", and the "person who is compulsive" can be named the "Minister for Perfectionism" etc.

Come to stay

As proposed above, methods involving therapeutic greetings can be used to announce the following. "Tell your frontal brain lobe what your cerebellum has already long understood: what you are feeling now has come to stay!"[4]

Since this does not invite a "yes, but" on the part of the client, her unconscious accepts the sentence as valid and the therapeutic outcome as long-lasting.[5]

The lonely symptom

The therapist can also work with provocative questions such as the following.

"I'm afraid that it will be very difficult to retrieve your symptom. Will you be very sad if I can't manage it?" … "But won't you miss it?" … "What will you do if you want your symptom again for some reason or other, and you can't find it any more?" … "What about if the symptom is sad and misses you, will you invite it over so that you can comfort it for a while?" … "Shouldn't I be worried about your symptom? Perhaps it's lonely, all on its own like that, without you?"… "You don't seem to be missing your symptom. Isn't it hard for you with it being gone like that?"

Ordeal

If it seems as though the client is sticking tenaciously to a behaviour or experience that she wants to be rid of according to what she actually says, use can be made of a particular form of therapeutic double bind for which Milton Erickson coined the term "ordeal" (order and deal).[6]

"There's a sure-fire way that you can achieve your objective with guaranteed success. At first glance it might not seem like an attractive proposal, but if you examine it very closely and think about what will happen, it's a straightforward and safe way of getting where you want to go. Would you like me to tell you how it works?" "Yes …" "Let's agree the following with each other, right now by shaking hands solemnly and later by confirming it in writing: for every cigarette that you smoke from now on (or any other undesired behaviour as appropriate), you must donate five euros to the political party you hate the most. Then you must go to the nearest bank to pay in the money, get a receipt and email a photo of it to me and to your five closest friends." "I'm not sure..." "Look at it this way: what's the chance that you'll continue to smoke if we reach this agreement?" "Zero." "Then you won't have to pay the penalty. Deal?"

If the client consents, the therapist notes down the key points of the agreement (what, how, from when, until when …) and ensures that the client has absolutely no desire or otherwise any opportunity to talk herself out of it, either before or after breaking the agreement. It can also be arranged that the client will send the therapist the exact wording of the agreement by the following day, and that the agreement will be renegotiated if anything is unclear. What matters is that the penalty is significantly more unpleasant than continuing the undesired behaviour. Donations to the children's home or a present of champagne for the therapist will not necessarily satisfy this criterion.

9.2 Scheduling appointments

There are no questions without implications, and that also applies to questions about the next session. If the therapist asks, "When should we meet again?", he implies that there is no possibility whatsoever that another session might not even be needed. If he asks, "Should we schedule another session?" or "Would you like us to schedule a follow-up session?", he implies that it might be the case that no further session is needed, while at the same time perhaps also expressing a preference for scheduling a follow-up session. I find it important to avoid any nocebo effect in relation to the duration of therapy as a result of such implications, and prefer instead to generate the expectation of a rapidly advancing process.

Confirming and cancelling a therapy session at short notice

"We have two options: we can schedule our next session, and you can cancel it or postpone it shortly beforehand if you find you don't need it after all, or you can leave it a few days and then email me to tell me whether you'd like another session, and if so when. Which would you prefer?"

Therapy session only when required

"As far as I'm concerned, we don't need to schedule another session on a particular date. Just get in touch with me if you need or want one. Would you be happy with that?"

Therapy session as a spa day

"I once had a client who left long gaps between her sessions with me. She told me that her acquaintances were always surprised when she told them that she looked forward to her therapy sessions. She said that for her it was like treating herself to a spa day."

Therapy session as a deployment by the fire brigade

"If there's ever an emergency of any kind whatsoever, you can call on me in the same way that you'd call on the fire brigade if there was a fire."

Therapy sessions as a safety net

"We can schedule our sessions together a bit like a safety net, which you only use if you need it. If we find out that you don't need any therapy or only need a little bit of therapy, we'll be done after quarter of an hour or half an hour, and I'll only bill you for the time that we spend together. If I end up with a gap in my schedule, I'll catch up on my paperwork."

Therapy session as a piano lesson

"We can arrange short appointments lasting only quarter of an hour or half an hour. You can tell me what's up with you, and I'll give you my thoughts and set you a few practical tasks that I think will help you to solve the problems. During the next session you can tell me how you got on with the exercises, what worked well and what we should tackle next. I'll share a few of my thoughts again, and suggest one, two, or three more exercises for you to try out. It'll work a bit like piano lessons; you practice at home, come here and perform to me, I suggest a few corrections and refinements, and then you go home and practice again until the next lesson."

Therapy session as a paradoxical intervention

A client who had previously suffered from the compulsive fear that one of her family members might become seriously ill still came to see me intermittently owing to "relapses". Once she told me, "Sometimes I have these relapses. They last for two or three days. Then my husband asks me, 'Why don't you visit your therapist?' And I answer, 'Good point – I'll call him tomorrow.' But by the following day my worries have vanished. Then I monitor the situation for a while with the aim of calling you as soon as they return, but they stay away." "Let's reach an agreement," I said to her. "On any working day, at any half-way normal time, you can hop into your car and come and ring on my doorbell. I promise you that if I'm not currently busy, we can hold a therapy session there and then, and otherwise we'll arrange for you to have the next free appointment, if possible on the same day. Do you agree with that?" The woman agreed. That was the last time I saw her, and years have passed since then.

Radiating a spirit of optimism

I typically give the signal that it is time to say goodbye with a certain level of buoyancy that expresses optimism about the positive developments that will emerge over the days and weeks to come. Exactly what this looks like depends on what has happened during the session and the frame of mind of the client and therapist, which makes generalisations impossible. Possible segues include the following.

"I believe that means that we're done! What do you think?"

"And so it's about time for us to bid farewell until next time, right?"
  "I'm looking forward to hearing how it goes!"
  "Let's see what happens now! I'm excited to hear!"
  "It's the start of a new era!"

9.3 Opening of the following session

How should the following session start? And how about the third, fourth, and fifth session? Can the therapist start each session in the same way as the first, or should something else be added?

Generally speaking, the therapist can ask the client how things have gone since the last session and how things should go in future, or in other words what is currently concerning the client. Generally speaking, it is safe for the therapist to stick to the rule that, "every session is a first session". The therapist can begin every session with the same question, for example: "Assuming that that this session went as well as it possibly could do and even better, what will have changed afterwards?" The therapist can also say something along the lines of the following. "If I may, I'd like to pretend that this is our first session, and ask you the following question: 'From where you're sitting now, what in your life needs to improve most (or most urgently)?'" Even if the therapist does not know all the details about the client's situation, he can ask: "What do you think we should definitely cover today? What do we want to explore together?"

9.4 Feedback on developments since the last session

It goes without saying that the therapist can also ask the client for guidance as follows.

"Would you like to update me on your situation?"

"Has anything got better or worse since last time? Has anything changed or stayed the same?"

Celebrating successes

If the client subsequently reports improvements, this should be viewed as a reason to celebrate.

> Progress ... should be "loaded with significance" to a high degree, i.e. particular importance should be attached to it ... The therapist should ask immediately whether it would be a good idea to do more of the same in order to build on this development. Yet the therapist should also enquire straight away, as a precaution, about any potential ambivalences (anticipating). This allows therapists and counsellors to escape the projection of constantly being agents of one-sided change ... The conclusion should be ... "celebrated". As a result, not only clients' contributions but also therapists' contributions are honoured appropriately. This is the best possible way of supporting future development on both sides![7]

The therapist can communicate his joy and (where applicable) his astonishment at the outcome.

"Great! I'm delighted for you!"

"Wow! How did you manage that!"

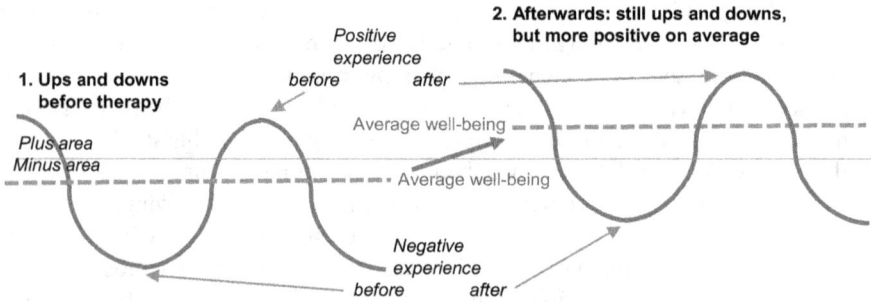

Figure 9.1 Ups and downs of life before and after therapy

"It seems to me like we won't need to see each other for much longer …"
"Now that's a reason to celebrate! How *could* you celebrate that?"

Evaluating setbacks

Conversely, if the client reports that things got worse for her after the therapy session, it's possible to discuss the following with her:

- when things started to get worse,
- what (probably) triggered this process,
- what impact the same event would have had prior to the last session.

The client generally reaches the conclusion that there was a triggering event. The question about whether this triggering event might have resulted in the client feeling even worse prior to the last therapy session is almost always answered in the affirmative, with astonishing clarity.

The therapist can make the client aware that the objective of therapy cannot be for her to avoid experiencing the ups and downs of life, but must instead be an upward shift in her average state of well-being. A drawing such as the following can be used for this purpose.

Initially (**1.**), the client's attitude to life is located predominantly in the minus area. Later (**2.**), it is located primarily in the plus area. Pleasant or stressful events lead to highs and lows afterwards just as they did before, but the highs are subsequently higher and the lows are not as low as before. The client's average well-being (dashed lines) has shifted upwards (Figure 9.1).

Clients frequently describe their state of mind since the last session by saying something along the lines of the following: "I felt OK for three days, but then I felt worse again." Enquiries reveal that the client's state of mind was nowhere near as bad as it had been prior to the therapy session – it was simply worse than it had been immediately after the session. A number of clients (usually those who prepare themselves for the following session in their thoughts) report that they felt better immediately before the therapy session. What might explain this phenomenon?

The subconscious is forced to select from a choice of many millions when choosing the memories from which it generates expectations. It therefore sorts through these memories based on the significance it assigns to them in terms of generating predictions of the future. In order to do so, it prioritises them on the basis of several different criteria:

- the *intensity (INT)* of the experience (trauma),
- the frequency and *duration (DUR)* of the experience (chronicity)
- the *topicality (TOP)* of something new that manifestly replaces something old (update remains an update, dead remains dead).

The latter is of central importance in terms of the effectiveness of the therapy. The intensity of perception and emotion and the perceived plausibility at the end of the session determine the strength of this factor, or in other words the stability of the outcome or the sustainability of therapy.[8]

If, a few hours after the therapy session, the client is feeling better than she felt before, she expects that this will also be the case for the next few sessions, and this is indeed what happens, because the expectation manifests itself as experience. After three good sessions she expects another three good sessions, and after one good day she expects another one. The memory of therapy fades after a few days, and with it the "hope" criterion of topicality. As a result, the client pays more attention to the intensity and duration of previous (negative) memories in order to generate expectations.

The diagram shows how a positive expectation (hope, arrows pointing upwards), obtained from relevant new memories of therapy, can – like a vector – be added to or subtracted from negative expectations (fear, from intense or durable biographical memories), and how the graph of well-being moves upwards or downwards over time (Figure 9.2).[9]

At Point 1 (after the first session), the positive expectation from the current (TOP1) positive memory predominates, and generates a high level of well-being. The positive expectation later fades (TOP2) and the level of well-being drops, while negative expectations are generated again from memories of intense (INT) or durable (DUR) negative experiences. The expectation of the next therapy session is generated from the memory of the preceding session, and so the level of well-being before the session improves as a result of current therapy memories being refreshed (TOP3).

Although the client might therefore have the feeling that she is suffering "relapses", she is actually progressing well. The therapist can point out that this is a typical pattern, that the overall trend is upwards and that she will achieve his objective if she "keeps on keeping on" (Figure 9.3).

If clients express disappointment that the positive outcome did not last for long, I sometimes explain this progression to them using a sketch, by drawing an arrow pointing upwards (right on the diagram) and telling them: "Upwards can also look like this!"

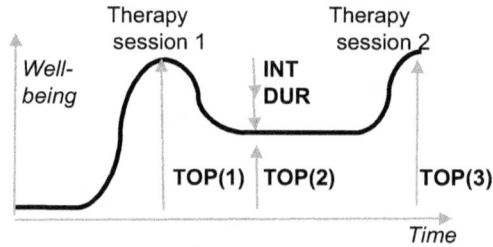

Figure 9.2 Development of well-being after therapy when new positive memories and expectations fade

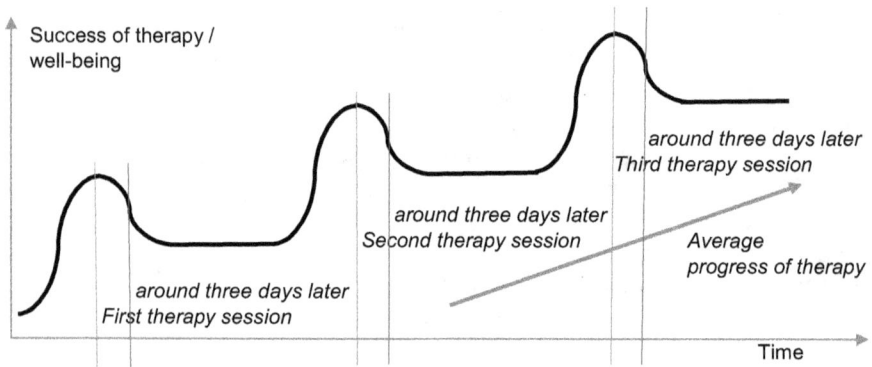

Figure 9.3 Development of well-being over a series of therapy sessions

Vineyard instead of rice terrace

The following explanation can then be provided:

"This is a rice terrace model. We can probably also turn it into a vineyard model. That would look like this … It works if your internal self generates expectations less and less on the basis of what was previously the case, and instead more and more consistently on the basis of what we are experiencing right now. In order to ensure that this is the case, it's a good idea for your internal self to appoint to posts within the Ministry of Confidence and Optimism more and more of the people who have perhaps still been cautious up until now and raised objections in order to protect you against disappointment" (Figure 9.4).

Announcing the unconscious effects of practice

"… Give a greeting to your internal self and tell it that what we are discovering will become even stronger from one session to the next as a result of the unconscious effects of practice …"

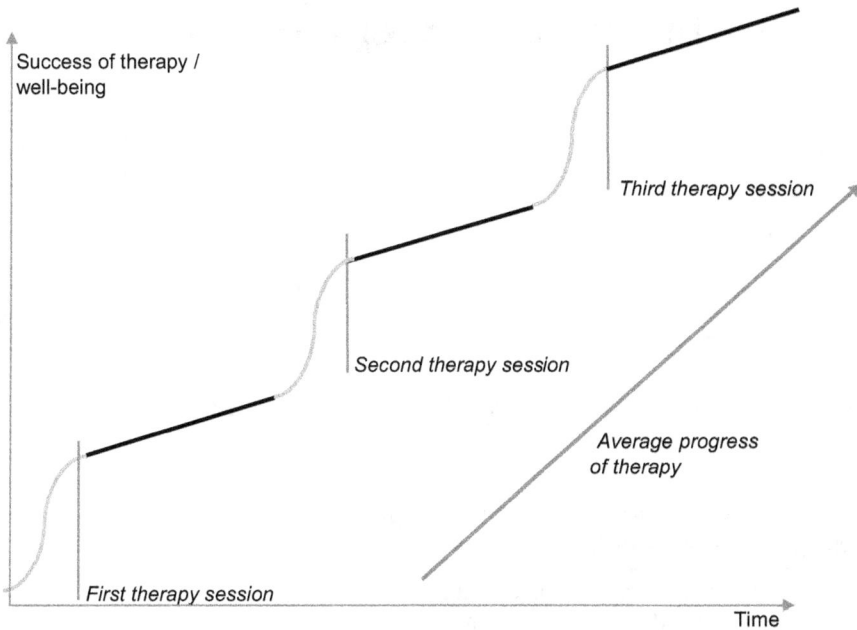

Figure 9.4 Development of well-being with full positive expectation (no scepticism) on the client's side

From the bud to the blossom

"… just like a rose that starts as a bud and then unfurls and in the process becomes even larger and more beautiful than it already was at the beginning. What do you think about that?"

Notes

1 See Chapter 2, section on hypnotherapy, "Factors affecting therapy", Factor 3, and "The cycle of memory and expectation".
2 Wense 2005, Werke 2, 958; see Hammel 2014a, 92 *et seq.*
3 Hammel 2020, 31.
4 See Hammel 2019a, 133f.
5 See Chapter 6 and Chapter 8, section "Therapeutic greetings".
6 For further details of the ordeal see von Schlippe & Schweitzer 1996, 197 *et seq.*; Hammel 2019a, 246; Hammel 2011, 271.
7 Schmidt 2005, 122 *et seq.*
8 See Factors 1 and 2 in Chapter 2, section on hypnotherapy, "Factors affecting therapy".
9 Prior 2006 refers to the fact that positive expectations regularly generate improvements even before the first therapy session.

List of individual interventions

Bibliography

Alman, B., & Lambrou, P. (1999). *Self-Hypnosis: The Complete Guide to better Health and Self-Change*. London: Routledge.

Alz, S. (2022). *Depression entschlüsseln: Ursachen verstehen und Lösungen finden*. Stuttgart: Klett-Cotta.

Balon, R. (2006). Mood, anxiety, and physical illness: Body and mind, or mind and body? *Depress Anxiety*, *23*(6), 377–387.

Bandler, R., & Grinder, J. (1981). *Trance-formations: Neurolinguistic Programming and the Structure of Hypnosis*. Boulder, CO: Real People.

Bartl, R. (2016). *Sucht, Angst, Zwang, Essstörungen. Hypnosystemische Perspektiven zum hilfreichen Umgang mit leidvollen Störungen und deren geschützten Anliegen*. C-Seminar Klinische Hypnose, Vienna: Hypno-Synstitut.

Bible (2011). *New International Version*. London: Hodder & Stoughton.

Beaulieu, D. (2006). *Impact Techniques for Therapists*. London: Routledge.

Bierman, S. (2020) *Healing Beyond Pills and Potions. Core Principles for Helpers and Healers*. Del Mar, CA: Gyro Press International.

Bierbaum-Luttermann, H., & Mrochen, S. (2019). *Klinische Hypnose und Hypnotherapie mit Kindern und Jugendlichen*. Paderborn: Junfermann.

Coan, J., Schaefer, H. & Davidson, R. (2006). Lending a hand: Social regulation of the neural response to threat. *Psychological Science*, *17*(12), 1032–1039. https://doi.org/10.1111/j.1467-9280.2006.01832.x.

Dietrich, D. (2016). *So gelingen Veränderungen! Mit hypnosystemischen Lösungen werden, wer Sie sein können*. Göttingen: Vandenhoeck.

Domanski, J.-O. (2022). *Worte, die wirken: Einführung in die hypnosystemische Seelsorge*. Gütersloh: Gütersloher Verlag.

Dunbar, R. (1997). *Grooming, Gossip, and the Evolution of Language*. London: Faber & Faber.

Eibl-Eibesfeldt, I. (1997). *Die Biologie des menschlichen Verhaltens: Grundriss der Humanethologie* (3rd ed.). Weyarn: Blank.

Erickson, M. (1959). Further clinical techniques of hypnosis: Utilisation techniques. *American Journal of Clinical Hypnotherapy*, *2*, 3–21.

Erickson, M., & Rossi, E. (1979). *Hypnotherapy: An Exploratory Casebook*. New York: Irvington.

Erickson, M., & Rossi, E. (1981). *Experiencing Hypnosis: Therapeutic Approaches to Altered States by Milton Erickson*. New York: Irvington.

Erickson, M., Rossi, E., & Rossi, S. (1976). *Hypnotic Realities: The Introduction of Clinical Hypnosis and Indirect Forms of Suggestion.* New York: Irvington.

Fritzsche, K., & Hartman, W. (2010). *Einführung in die Ego-State-Therapie.* Heidelberg: Carl-Auer.

Fritzsche, K. (2013). *Praxis der Ego-State-Therapie.* Heidelberg: Carl-Auer.

Fruth, S. (2021). *Imaginäre Körperreisen: Neue Wege zum individuellen Heilungsprozess.* Heidelberg: Carl Auer.

Gapp, K., Bohacek, J., Grossmann, J., Brunner, A., Manuella, F., Nanni, P., & Mansuy, I. (2016): Potential of Environmental Enrichment to Prevent Transgenerational Effects of Paternal Trauma, *Neuropsychopharmacology, 41,* 2749–2758.

Goodwin, R., Galea, S., Perzanowski, M., & Jacobi, F. (2012): Impact of allergy treatment on the association between allergies and mood and anxiety in a population sample. *Clinical and Experimental Allergy, 42*(12), 1765–1771. https://doi.org/ 10.1111/j.1365–2222.2012.04042.x.

Gordon, D., & Meyers-Anderson, M. (2018). *Phoenix: Therapeutic Patterns of Milton H. Erickson.* Tucson, AZ: David Gordon.

Groß, M., & Popper, V. (2020). *Und die Maus hört ein Rauschen: Hypnosystemisches Erleben in Therapie, Coaching und Beratung. (Reden reicht nicht!?)* Heidelberg: Carl Auer.

Häublein, P. (2018). *Hypnosystemische Konzepte zum Umgang mit Prüfungsangst bei Studierenden.* Heidelberg: Carl Auer.

Haley, J. (1993). *Uncommon Therapy. The Psychiatric Techniques of Milton H. Erickson, M.D.* New York: Norton.

Haley, J. (2011). *Ordeal-Therapy: Unusual Ways to Change Behavior.* Bancyfelin: Crown House.

Hammel, S. (2009). Tinnitustherapie durch Hypnose: Der Heidelberger Pilotversuch. *Musica Sacra, 4*(9), 223–226.

Hammel, S. (2010). Von Möwenfelsen und Felsenbirnen: Aufbruchsgeschichten für Kinder und Jugendliche. *Familiendynamik, 2,* 136–143.

Hammel, S. (2011). *Handbuch der therapeutischen Utilisation: Vom Nutzen des Unnützen in Psychotherapie, Kinder- und Familientherapie, Heilkunde und Beratung.* Stuttgart: Klett-Cotta.

Hammel, S. (2012a). Metapher. In: Kleve, H. & Wirth, J. (Eds.), *Lexikon des systemischen Arbeitens: Grundbegriffe der Systemischen Praxis, Methodik und Theorie.* Heidelberg: Carl Auer, 264–267.

Hammel, S. (2012b). Utilisation. In: Kleve, H., Wirth, J. (Eds.): *Lexikon des systemischen Arbeitens: Grundbegriffe der Systemischen Praxis, Methodik und Theorie.* Heidelberg: Carl Auer, 441–444.

Hammel, S. (2012c). *The Blade of Grass in the Desert: Storytelling: Forgotten Medicine for Healing the Soul. A Story of 100 Stories for Counselling and Therapy.* Mainz: Impress.

Hammel, S. (2014a). *Therapie zwischen den Zeilen: Das ungesagt Gesagte in Beratung, Therapie und Heilkunde.* Stuttgart: Klett-Cotta.

Hammel, S. (2014b). *Das Sofa des Glücks. Therapeutisches Modellieren mit Paaren: Video documentation of a seminar at the Future Congress in Abano Terme.* Müllheim: Auditorium.

Hammel, S. (2015). *The Island of Love: A Game for Couple Therapy.* Kaiserslautern: hsb westpfalz.

Hammel, S. (2016a). *Alles neu gerahmt! Psychische Symptome in ungewöhnlicher Perspektive.* Munich: Ernst Reinhardt.

Hammel, S. (2016b). *Loslassen und leben. Befreiende Geschichten.* Mainz: Impress.

Hammel, S. (2016c). Utilisation – Wie spanne ich das Problem vor die Karre der Lösung? Video documentation of a seminar at the IGST in Heidelberg, hsb westpfalz.

Hammel, S. (2018a). *The Art of Therapeutic Storytelling.* Audio recording (CD/stream) of an introductory workshop seminar in collaboration with BSMDH Scotland. Kaiserslautern, hsb westpfalz.

Hammel, S. (2018b) *Therapeutic Modeling in Couple Therapy.* Video recording on the 2nd International Festival of Therapeutic Storytelling. Kaiserslautern, hsb westpfalz.

Hammel, S. (2019a). *Handbook of Therapeutic Storytelling: Stories and Metaphors in Psychotherapy, Child and Family Therapy, Medical Treatment, Coaching and Supervision.* Routledge: London.

Hammel, S. (2019b). *Lebensmöglichkeiten entdecken: Veränderung durch Therapeutisches Modellieren.* Stuttgart: Klett-Cotta.

Hammel, S. (2020). *Therapeutic Interventions in Three Sentences: Reshaping Ericksonian Hypnotherapy by Talking to the Brain and Body.* London: Routledge.

Hammel, S. (2024). *Therapeutisches Erzählen Lernen: Das Wichtigste in Kürze.* Berlin: Springer Nature.

Hammel, S., Hürzeler, A., Lamprecht, K., & Niedermann, M. (2015). *Wie das Krokodil zum Fliegen kam: 120 Geschichten, die das Leben verändern.* Munich: Ernst Reinhardt.

Hammel, S., Hürzeler, A., Lamprecht, K., & Niedermann, M. (2018). *Wie der Bär zum Tanzen kam: 120 Geschichten für einen gesunden Körper.* Munich: Ernst Reinhardt.

Hammel, S., Hürzeler, A., Lamprecht, K., & Niedermann, M. (2021). *Wie der Tiger lieben lernte: 120 Geschichten zum Umgang mit psychischem Trauma.* Munich: Ernst Reinhardt.

Hammel, S., Hürzeler, A., Lamprecht, K., & Niedermann M. (2023). *Wie das Nashorn Freiheit fand: 120 Geschichten zum Umgang mit Krisen.* Munich: Ernst Reinhardt.

Hammel, S., Vlamynck, A., & Weinspach, C. (2020). Ängste entzaubern, Lebensfreude finden: Die besten Interventionen aus 9 Therapierichtungen. Stuttgart: Klett-Cotta.

Hammond, C. (Ed.) (1990). *Handbook of Hypnotic Suggestions and Metaphors.* New York: Norton.

Harari, Y. (2011). *Sapiens: A Brief History of Humankind.* London: Penguin.

Hellinger, B. (1994). *Ordnungen der Liebe: Ein Kurs-Buch.* Heidelberg: Carl-Auer.

Herz, M. (2010). *Alte Heilgebete: Gesundheit für Körper und Geist.* Munich: Nymphenburger.

Hesse, P. (2003). *Teilearbeit. Konzepte von Multiplizität in ausgewählten Bereichen moderner Psychotherapie.* Heidelberg: Carl-Auer.

Holmes, T., & Holmes, I. (2007). *Reisen in die Innenwelt: Systemische Arbeit mit Persönlichkeitsanteilen.* Munich: Kösel.

Holtz, K., Mrochen, S., Nemetschek, P., & Trenkle, B. (Eds.) (2000). *Neugierig aufs Großwerden: Praxis der Hypnotherapie mit Kindern und Jugendlichen.* Heidelberg: Carl Auer.

Hullmann, I. (2020). Psychologie der Leichtigkeit: *In 5 Schritten Wahrnehmungsperspektive und Bewusstsein erweitern.* Stuttgart: Schattauer.

Hullmann, I. (2023). *Hypnosystemische Top-10-Tools: Mit Leichtigkeit wirksam werden in Therapie und Coaching.* Stuttgart, Schattauer.

Kachler, R. (2010). *Hypnosystemische Trauerbegleitung. Ein Leitfaden für die Praxis.* Heidelberg: Carl Auer.

Kachler, R. (2015). *Die Therapie des Paar-Unbewussten: Ein tiefenpsychologisch-hypnosystemischer Ansatz.* Munich: Klett-Cotta.

Kachler, R. (2018). *Nachholende Trauerarbeit: Hypnosystemische Beratung und Therapie bei frühen Verlusten.* Heidelberg: Carl Auer.

Kachler, R. (2021a). *Traumatische Verluste: Hypnosystemische Arbeit mit traumatisierten Trauernden. Ein Leitfaden für die Praxis.* Heidelberg: Carl Auer. [AQ'd Ch3]

Kachler, R. (2021b). *Kinder im Verlustschmerz begleiten: Hypnosystemische, traumafundierte Trauerarbeit mit Kindern und Jugendlichen.* Stuttgart: Klett-Cotta.

Kluschatzka-Valera, R. (2022). *Hypnosystemisches Case Management in der Sozialen Arbeit. Unterstützungssituationen gestalten.* Heidelberg: Carl Auer.

Kolodej, C. (2016). *Strukturaufstellungen für Konflikte, Mobbing und Mediation: Vom sichtbaren Unsichtbaren.* Berlin: Springer Nature.

Korzybski, A. (1994). *Science and Sanity: An Introduction to Non-Aristotelian Systems and General Semantics* (5th ed.). New York: Institute of General Semantics (1st ed.: 1933).

Lamprecht, Katharina (2020). *Die Rennschildkröte: 31 therapeutische Geschichten für Kinder.* Munich: Ernst Reinhardt.

Lang, A. (2022*). Konstruktivistische Psychotherapie Prozess-Hypno-Systemisch: Das Bonner Ressourcen Modell.* Munich: Elsevier

Leeb, W., Trenkle, B., & Weckenmann, M. (2011). *Der Realitätenkellner: Hypnosystemische Konzepte in Beratung, Coaching und Supervision.* Heidelberg: Carl Auer.

Lieberman, M., Inagaki, T., Tabibie, G., & Crockett, M. (2011). Subjective responses to emotional stimuli during labeling, reappraisal, and distraction, *Emotion* 11(3), 468–80. https://doi.org/10.1037/a0023503.

Mansuy, I., Gurret, J.-M., & Lefief-Delcourt, A. (2020). *Wir können unsere Gene steuern! Die Chancen der Epigenetik für ein gesundes und glückliches Leben.* Berlin: Berlin Verlag.

Maurer, A. (2021). Voice of Paul Watzlawick in an interview in 1981. Radiokolleg, part 4: *Paul Watzlawick, an optimistic nihilist,* in: ORF radio emission on 29 July 2021.

Meiss, O. (2016). *Hypnosystemische Therapie bei Depression und Burnout.* Heidelberg: Carl Auer.

Meyer-Erben, C., & Zander-Schreindorfer, U. (2021). *Hypnosystemisch arbeiten: Ein kleiner Praxisleitfaden.* Göttingen: Vandenhoeck.

Molcho, S. (1994). *Körpersprache.* Munich: Mosaik.

Mücke, K. (1998). *Probleme sind Lösungen: Systemische Beratung und Psychotherapie – ein pragmatischer Ansatz. Lehr- und Lernbuch.* Potsdam: Ökosysteme.

Muffler, E. (Ed.) (2015). *Kommunikation in der Psychoonkologie: Der hypnosystemische Ansatz.* Heidelberg: Carl Auer.

Nemetschek, P. (2006). *Systemische Familientherapie mit Kindern, Jugendlichen und Eltern: Lebensfluss-Modelle und analoge Methoden.* Stuttgart: Klett-Cotta.

Niedrist, A. (2019). *Wenn Scham und Beschämung das Leben behindern: Wie verändert sich die Scham unter hypnosystemischer Beratung?* Beau Bassin: Lehrbuchverlag.

O'Hanlon, H., & Hexum, A. (1990). *An Uncommon Casebook: The Complete Clinical Work of Milton H. Erickson, M.D.* New York: Norton.

Olness, K., & Kohen, D. (2011*). Hypnosis and Hypnotherapy with Children.* London: Routledge.

Pascal, B. (1961). *Pensées.* London, Penguin.

Peichl, J. (2019). *Einführung in die hypnosystemische Teiletherapie.* Heidelberg: Carl Auer.

Peichl, J. (2022). *Jedes Ich ist viele Teile: Die inneren Selbst-Anteile als Ressource nutzen.* Munich: Kösel.

Peyton, S. (2017). *Your Resonant Self: Guided Meditations and Exercises to Engage Your Brain's Capacity for Healing.* New York: Norton.

Peyton, S. (2021). *Your Resonant Self Workbook: From Self-sabotage to Self-care.* New York: Norton.

Pfeifer, P. (2019). *Hypnosystemische Beratung: Hypnosystemisches Menschenbild im nicht freiwilligen Kontext*. Munich: Grin.

Prior, M. (2006). Beratung und Therapie optimal vorbereiten: Informationen und Interventionen vor dem ersten Gespräch. Heidelberg: Carl Auer.

Prior, M. (2017). *MiniMax Interventions: 15 Simple Therapeutic Interventions That Have Maximum Impact*. Bancyfelin: Crown House.

Reinhardt, M. (2018). *Systemische Pädagogik und Beratung*. Präsentation im Aufbaukurs Heidelberg: Helm-Stierlin-Institut.

Rießbeck H. (2013). *Einführung in die hypnodynamische Teiletherapie*. Heidelberg: Carl Auer.

Rosen, S. (Ed.) (1982). *My Voice Will Go with You: The Teaching Tales of Milton H. Erickson*. New York: Norton.

Roy-Byrne, P., Davidson, K., Kessler, R., Asmundson, G., Goodwin, R., Kubzansky, L., Lydiard, R., Massie, M., Katon, W., Laden, S., & Stein, M. (2008). Anxiety disorders and comorbid medical illness. *General Hospital Psychiatry*, *30*, 208–225.

Saint-Exupéry, A. de (2017). *The Little Prince*. London: Egmont.

Satir, V. (2018): Kommunikation ist ein riesiger Regenschirm … der alles umfasst, was unter Menschen vor sich geht. Munich: Klett-Cotta.

Schlippe, A. von, & Schweitzer J. (1996). *Lehrbuch der systemischen Beratung*. Göttingen: Vandenhoeck.

Schmidt, G. (2004). *Liebesaffären zwischen Problem und Lösung: Hypnosystemisches Arbeiten in schwierigen Kontexten*. Heidelberg: Carl Auer.

Schmidt, G. (2005). *Einführung in die Hypnosystemische Therapie und Beratung*. Heidelberg: Carl Auer.

Schmidt, G. (2009). *Von der Psychosomatik zur Somatopsychik: Für achtungsvolle, Kompetenz-aktivierende Hypnotherapie bei als körperlich erlebten Beschwerden (wie z. B. Fybromyalgie, Allergien u. a.)*. Video documentation, Müllheim: Auditorium

Schmidt, G., Dollinger, A., & Müller-Kalthoff, B. (Eds.) (2010). *Gut beraten in der Krise: Konzepte und Werkzeuge für ganz alltägliche Ausnahmesituationen*. Bonn: managerSeminare.

Schneider, P. (2009). Musik, von Engeln vorgesungen: Entstehung und Ursachen von Tinnitus und Geräuschempfindlichkeit bei Kirchenmusikern, Chorleitern, Bläsern und Sängern. *Musica Sacra*, *4*(9), 220–222.

Schneider, P., Andermann, M., Wengenroth, M., Goebel, R., Flor, H., Rupp, A., & Diesch, E. (2009). Reduced volume of Heschl's gyrus in tinnitus. *Neuroimage*, *45*, 927–939.

Schulz von Thun, F. (1998). *Miteinander reden 3: Das Innere Team und situationsgerechte Kommunikation*. Reinbek: Rowohlt.

Schulz von Thun, F., & Stegemann, W. (Eds.) (2004). *Das innere Team in Aktion: Praktische Arbeit mit dem Modell*. Reinbek: Rowohlt.

Schwartz, R. (2003). *Systemische Therapie mit der inneren Familie*. Stuttgart: Klett-Cotta.

Schweitzer, J., & Schlippe, A. von (2007). *Lehrbuch der systemischen Therapie und Beratung II: Das störungsspezifische Wissen*. Göttingen: Vandenhoeck.

Seemann, H. (2022). *Schmerzen – Notrufe aus dem Körper: Hypnosystemische Schmerztherapie*. Stuttgart: Klett-Cotta.

Sellam, S. (2006). *Les allergies: C'est plus simple qu'on le pense*. Montreuil-Bonnin: bérangel.

Shazer, S. de, Dolan, Y., with Korman, H., Trepper, T., McCollum, E., & Berg, I.K.

(2021). *More Than Miracles: The State of the Art of Solution-Focused Brief Therapy.* London: Routledge.

Short, D., & Weinspach, C. (2007). *Hoffnung und Resilienz: Therapeutische Strategien von Milton H. Erickson.* Heidelberg: Carl Auer.

Signer-Fischer, S. (2022). *Schlafhund, Schutzanzug & Co.: Hypnosystemische Methoden zur Unterstützung der jugendlichen Entwicklung.* Heidelberg: Carl Auer.

Simon, F., & Rech-Simon, C. (2000). *Zirkuläres Fragen – Systemische Therapie in Fallbeispielen: Ein Lernbuch.* Heidelberg: Carl Auer.

Spork, P. (2017). *Gesundheit ist kein Zufall – Wie das Leben unsere Gene prägt: Die neuesten Erkenntnisse der Epigenetik.* München: DVA.

Starker, V., & Peschke, T. (2017). *Hypnosystemische Perspektiven im Change Management: Veränderung steuern in einer volatilen, komplexen und widersprüchlichen Welt.* Berlin: Springer Nature.

Stefano, A. de (2019). *"Ich habe einen Therapeuten gesucht und einen Realitätenkellner gefunden!": Die hypnosystemische Methode in der Praxis.* Oberpframmern: Neue Stadt.

Stone, S., & Stone, H. (1989*). Embracing Our Selves: The Voice Dialogue Manual.* Novato: New World.

Theuretzbacher, K., & Nemetschek, P. (2009). *Coaching und Systemische Supervision mit Herz, Hand und Verstand: Handlungsorientiert arbeiten, Systeme aufbauen.* Stuttgart: Klett-Cotta.

Unterberger, G., Wilcke, I., & Witt, K. (2014). *Allergien mental behandeln – Damit Geist und Körper wieder angemessen reagieren können: Modelle und Strategien angewandter Psychoneuroimmunologie.* Bargteheide: Psymed.

Varga von Kibéd, M., & Sparrer, I. (2000). *Ganz im Gegenteil: Tetralemmaarbeit und andere Grundformen Systemischer Strukturaufstellungen – für Querdenker und solche, die es werden wollen.* Heidelberg: Carl Auer.

Velasco Valenzuela Vázquez, G. de (2020). *ABC of Solution-focused Systemic Structural Constellations: Learn to constellate in the most practical and resolute way through the transverbal language of Matthias Varga von Kibéd and Insa Sparrer.* Independently published.

Vlamynck, A. (2019). *Klopfen für die Selbstwertstärkung: Wie Energetische Psychologie hilft.* Stuttgart: Klett-Cotta.

Wall, P. (1982). *Die drei Phasen des Übels: Die Beziehung von Verletzung und Schmerz.* In: Keeser, W., Pöppel, E., & Mitterhusen, P. (Eds.), *Das Rätsel des Schmerzes.* München: Urban, 30–45.

Wallis, V. (1994). *Two Old Women: An Alaska Legend of Betrayal, Courage and Survival.* New York: Harper Collins

Watzlawick, P. (1976). *How Real Is Real? Confusion, Disinformation, Communication.* New York: Random House.

Watzlawick, P. (1978). *The Language of Change: Elements of Therapeutic Communication.* New York: Basic Books.

Watzlawick, P., Jackson, D., & Beavin Bavelas, J. (1967). *Pragmatics of Human Communication: A Study of Interactional Patterns, Pathologies and Paradoxes.* New York: Norton.

Watzlawick, P., Weakland, J., & Fisch, R. (2011). *Change: Principles of Problem Formation and Problem Resolution.* New York: Norton.

Weakland, J. (1960). The "Double-Bind" Hypothesis of Schizophrenia and Three-Party Interaction. In: Jackson, D. (Ed.), *The Etiology of Schizophrenia.* New York: Basic Books.

Weber, G. Schmidt, G., & Simon, F. (2005). *Aufstellungsarbeit revisited ... nach Hellinger?*. Heidelberg: Carl Auer.

Wense, H. von der (2005). *Von Aas bis Zylinder: Werke* (Eds. Niehoff, R. & Bertoncini, V.). Frankfurt am Main: Zweitausendeins.

Wetter, R. (2022). *Hypnosystemische Lebensberatung: Grundlagen und Impulse für die Praxis*. Göttingen: Vandenhoeck.

Witt, K. (2008). Neuro-Linguistic Psychotherapy (NLPt) treatment can modulate the reaction in pollen allergic humans and their state of health. *International Journal of Psychotherapy*, *12*(1), 50–60.

Wittgenstein L. (2001). *Tractatus logico-philosopicus*. London: Routledge

Yehuda, R., Daskalakis, N.P., Bierer, L.M., Bader, H.N., Klengel, T., Holsboer, F., & Binder, E.B. (2016). Holocaust exposure induced intergenerational effects on FKBP5 methylation. *Biological Psychiatry*, *80*(5), 372–380.

Zeig, J. (1985). *Experiencing Erickson: An Introduction to the Man and his Works*. New York: Brunner, Mazel.

Zeig, J. (Ed.) (1982). *Ericksonian Approaches to Hypnosis and Psychotherapy*. New York: Brunner.

Zeig, J. (Ed.) (1999). *A Teaching Seminar with Milton H. Erickson*. London: Routledge.

Ziegler, C., Grundner-Culemann, F., Schiele, M. A., Schlosser, P., Kollert, L., Mahr, M., Gajewska, A., Lesch, K.-P., Deckert, J., Köttgen, A., & Domschke, K. (2016). MAOA gene hypometylation in panic disorder: Reversability of an epigenetic risk pattern by psychotherapy. *Translational Psychiatry*, *6*, e773.

Index

For Product Safety Concerns and Information please contact our EU
representative GPSR@taylorandfrancis.com
Taylor & Francis Verlag GmbH, Kaufingerstraße 24, 80331 München, Germany

www.ingramcontent.com/pod-product-compliance
Lightning Source LLC
Chambersburg PA
CBHW050642280326
41932CB00015B/2744

'Stefan Hammel shows convincingly how his approach helps patients to transform their lives. In his helpful and informative book the author reveals the origin of his approach based on solid theoretical foundations which integrates systemic approach with ericksonian hypnosis reinforced by reflective practice aimed at highlighting what works best with different patients. This book is suitable for those who are curious to receive new insights and are ready to learn new ways of working with patients, experimenting a new interactive therapeutic approach also using therapeutic metaphors and stories, maps and landscapes, drawings and objects, space and rituals.'

Consuelo Casula, *Clinical Psychologist and Hypnotherapist, Former President of the European Society of Hypnosis, Recipient of the International Society of Hypnosis Pierre Janet Award for Clinical Excellence in 2022, Italy*

'This is not the type of book that you can just pick up and skim but it will surely reward you many times over for the time that you put into it. It is another major contribution from master storyteller Stefan Hammel, which has something in it for everyone. First and foremost, it provides a wonderful overview of hypnosystemic therapy, its history, the way in which it integrates with other schools of thought and most importantly how to do it. Contained within its pages are an incredible 160 therapeutic interventions. Perhaps best of all, there is an index telling you where to locate each of these interventions. So instead of trying to remember "Where was it I saw that great technique about "Tilling the Field" or "Turning Shit into Roses" you no longer have to spend hours pouring over the entire book– you can go straight to it. This book will not only help you transform the lives of your clients, it may well transform the way you do therapy.'

Brian Allen, *Psychologist, Chair of The Australian Society of Hypnosis Western Australia (ASH WA), Director of Training, ASH WA*

'Stefan encourages the therapist to be as flexible and diverse in their therapeutic approach as the patient sitting in front of them. The examples of real clients are excellent and make the outcomes seem readily achievable which will encourage the reader to feel positive about using these techniques. Stefan pays homage to his influencers and teachers, but while some of the techniques may be based on Paul Watzlawick and Milton Erickson the content is genuinely "Hammel."'

Dr Kathleen Long, *MBChB, MPH, DRCOG, NLP, Master Practitioner MBTI (level 1), Past President ESH, Past President BSMDH, Hon Chairperson BSMDH*

'Stefan Hammel has done it again. As with his previous works, he gives us a clear, accessible, theoretically sound, and very practical book of therapeutic wisdom. This is what we have come to expect from him. But this volume also transcends.

His rich explanation of hypno-systemic therapy not only provides a framework for insight into his many useful strategies and examples, but a platform for inspiring clinicians across the continuum of health and care to become more effective in their work. Hammel's new book is destined to become a well-worn resource.'

Laurence Irwin Sugarman, *MD, Research Professor, College of Health Sciences and Technology, Rochester Institute of Technology. Rochester, New York, USA. Author of* Changing Minds with Clinical Hypnosis: Narrative and Discourse for a New Health Care Paradigm.

'The resourceful guide, *Transforming Lives with Hypnosystemic Therapy*, offers a comprehensive exploration of hypno-systemic therapy, emphasizing effective application. Authored by a knowledgeable practitioner, Stefan Hammel, it provides valuable insights into therapeutic strategies and interventions beneficial for both novices and experienced practitioners in the field. The book is not only instructive but also enjoyable and inspiring, making it essential for anyone interested in the topic. Skillfully weaving in discussions on basic assumptions and foundations, this book is poised to become a crucial reference for therapy and coaching.'

Anita Jung, *LPC-S, LPA, Past President American Society of Clinical Hypnosis President, Central Texas Society of Clinical Hypnosis*